MEDARD BOSS AND THE PROMISE OF THERAPY

THE BEGINNINGS OF DASEINSANALYSIS

MILES GROTH

First published in 2020 by
Free Association Books

Copyright © 2020 Miles Groth

The author's rights are fully asserted. The rights of
Miles Groth to be identified as the author of this work
has been asserted by him in accordance with the
Copyright, Designs and Patents Act 1988

A CIP Catalogue of this book is available from
the British Library

ISBN: 978-1-91138-336-9

All rights reserved; no part of this publication may be reproduced,
stored in a retrieval system, or transmitted, in any form or by
any means, electronic, mechanical, photocopying, recording or
otherwise, without the prior written permission of the publisher.
Nor be circulated in any form of binding or cover other than that
in which it is published and a similar condition including this
condition being imposed on the subsequent purchaser.

Typeset by
Typo•glyphix
www.typoglyphix.co.uk

Cover design by
Candescent

Printed in the UK

Table of Contents

Preface	v
Contexts	1
Introduction	9
Problems of Terminology and Translation	12

Part I "Da-seinanalysis" in Print — 23

A. Early Publications Influenced by Martin Heidegger — 25

    1. Meaning and Content of the Sexual Perversions — 25
    2. Psychoanalysis and Daseinsanalysis — 52

B. The Two Dream Books — 61

    1. The Analysis of Dreams — 62
    2. "I dreamt last night..." — 64

C. The *magnum opus*: The *Existential Foundations of Medicine and Psychology* — 66

D. The Zollikon Seminars — 70

    1. *Zollikon Seminars: Protocols—Letters—Conversations* — 70
    2. The Two Editions of the *Zollikoner Seminare* — 72
        a. The Background of the *Gesamtausgabe* Edition of *Zollikoner Seminare* — 73
        b. Discrepancies between *GA 89* and the Boss Edition of the *Zollikoner Seminare* — 84

Table of Contents

Part II   A New Beginning for Therapy   97

A. Boss, Heidegger, and the East   99

   A Psychiatrist Discovers India   99

B. From "Da-seinanalysis" to Therapy   123

Concluding Thoughts   129

Appendices: Texts and Materials   131

Appendix I: "Vorwort" to the 2nd Edition of *Sinn und Gehalt der sexuellen Perversionen* (1952)   133

Appendix II: "Vorwort" to the 3rd Edition of *Sinn und Gehalt der sexuellen Perversionen* (1966)   135

Appendix III: "Nachwort" to the 3rd Edition of *Sinn und Gehalt der sexuellen Perversionen* (1966)   140

Appendix IV: A Comparison of the Table of Contents of the first (1947) and second (1952) editions of *Sinn und Gehalt der sexuellen Perversionen*   148

Appendix V: "Nachwort" to the 3rd Edition of *Indienfahrt eines Psychiaters* (1976)   154

Appendix A: Chart Comparing the Editions of the Zollikon Seminars   158

Appendix B: Tables of Contents of the Three Editions   162

Appendix C: Notes on Trawny's Manuscript Sources   193

Appendix D: Notes on the Boss Edition   195

An International Bibliography of the Writings of Medard Boss (1929-2003))   202

   Chronological List of Publications   237
   Thematic Index to the Chronological List of Publications   244
   Name Index   246

Glossary   247
Index   249

Preface

This is primarily a book of texts and materials for renewed study of the work of the Swiss psychiatrist Medard Boss (1903-1990). In it the reader will find translations of important texts by Boss not previously available in English. The present volume will be especially useful for English-speaking readers who might not have access to Boss's publications in German.

In 1987, Vittorio Klostermann published Martin Heidegger's *Zollikoner Seminare. Protokolle—Zwiegespräche—Briefe*, edited by Boss. Thirty years later, Heidegger's notes for the seminars were first published along with the previously published protocols as Volume 89 (*GA* 89, 2018) of the Heidegger *Complete Edition* [*Gesamtausgabe*], edited by Peter Trawny. The appearance of this volume calls for a look back at and reappraisal of Boss's edition and his legacy. The present work is a contribution to both. I believe Boss is among our best guides toward a genuinely human therapy.

There is no full-length biography of Boss and, sadly, we lack adequate English translations of his books and papers. A German collected edition has not yet been prepared and apart from two anthologies Boss published in his lifetime (1979, 1982), his many other papers are scattered in books and journals, some of them very difficult to track down. Although late in life he reluctantly founded a training institute in Switzerland, there is no school dedicated to his unique view of existential therapy and only a few individuals consider themselves to be in his tradition. As a result, he has no real "followers" and little has been written about his legacy.

My goal is to reacquaint counselors and psychotherapists and perhaps even a few psychiatrists with the ideas of this remarkable

Preface

figure in the history of twentieth-century psychology, someone who quietly but radically deviated from the mainstream of standard thinking and practice of his time.

A physician and psychoanalyst who knew Sigmund Freud, Eugen Bleuler, and Carl Gustav Jung, Medard Boss was also the only psychologist to have been in extended, close collegial and personal contact with the German thinker Martin Heidegger. In midlife he surprised his colleagues and friends by seeking out first-hand experiences of Eastern spiritual practices as a novice in relationships with several gurus in India where he had traveled to lecture and supervise psychiatrists.

Patrician, yet sporty, a dedicated physician but also a seeker, philosophically and spiritually, Boss was one of those fabled men who are ahead of their time. I hope this study will help bring him back into the present and perhaps, at last, his own time.

This book is also necessary, given the publication, in 2018, of Martin Heidegger's notes for the *Zollikon Seminars* he gave at Boss's home in Switzerland in the 1960s. Its appearance calls for revisiting Boss's own edition of the seminars published in 1987. I do this below in the context of Boss's earlier works influenced by Heidegger.

The present volume is offered in respectful observance of the thirtieth anniversary of the death of Medard Boss (1903-1990).

Contexts Mostly Personal

My interest in returning to the contribution of Medard Boss is the future of psychotherapy. I am concerned about what it has become and want to see it remain true to its original purpose, which I believe Boss understood better than anyone (except perhaps R.D. Laing) but could not fully realize in his own practice. I also want to bring to attention certain events in Boss's life that have not been sufficiently appreciated but deeply affected the development of his existential analysis.

Throughout I will emphasize the great difference between psychiatry and other medical specialties, on the one hand, which are devoted to the treatment of the human body's organic disorders, and *therapy*, which is directed at the human being's existence. Boss is unique in having been both a "real psychiatrist" and a "real therapist"—and a rebel in both groups. As a psychiatrist, for example, he continued to explore the psychosomatic hypothesis, even while psychiatry was busy rejecting it and embracing neuropsychology and psychopharmacology. As a psychotherapist, he abandoned some of the basic theoretical concepts of classic psychoanalysis such as transference in favor of an existential form of psychoanalysis—a form of psychoanalysis without the psyche.

I write as someone who, in the late 1960s, at the time when Boss's existential analysis was taking on its final form, out of personal need experienced my own psychoanalytic therapy with someone who, like Boss, was a psychiatrist and psychoanalyst, having completed psychoanalytic training in the 1950s at a nationally and internationally recognized medical psychoanalytic institute in the United States. Later, during the 1970s, I re-established contact with him and we worked together on theoretical and practical aspects of therapy. He became my mentor and friend.

In 1980, I moved to New York to prepare to provide psychoanalysis and psychoanalytic therapy since there were no lay analytic institutes where I lived. There I underwent a five-year-long training analysis at such an institute. I was supervised while seeing patients at two other lay institutes' outpatient services, at one of which I had first enrolled in its course of study in psychoanalytic psychotherapy. It was for me a period of intensive reading of the psychoanalytic literature. In 1982, I published a paper on Freud and Heidegger in the *International Review of Psycho-Analysis*.[1]

My initial commitment as a therapist, then, was to classic Freudian psychoanalysis, but it had been challenged from the start by my reading of Martin Heidegger's major work, *Being and Time*, which I had undertaken for the first time in 1968, the year I graduated from college.

To back up a little: I first heard about Heidegger in 1965. The year before that, I had been sent by my parents to a liberal arts college to prepare for medical school and a career as a physician. I turned my back on the "pre-med" curriculum, however, because the laboratory setting that was an essential part of studying biology and chemistry (the bedrock "pre-med" courses) seemed to me to have nothing to do with preparing me to care for people who were ill. I still believe it does not, although I later became interested in chemistry, primarily as the science responsible for investigating substances that have come to be known as having "psychotropic" properties, pharmaceuticals used extensively since about 1960 by psychiatrists in the treatment of so-called mental illnesses or diseases of the mind.

The year I heard about Heidegger, I declared a major in philosophy. Quite by chance, it happened that an errant professor in the philosophy department offered a special topics seminar on Maurice Merleau-Ponty's *Phenomenology of Perception*. This remarkable book introduced me to Jean-Paul Sartre and Heidegger, and Edmund Husserl, pretty much in that order.

---

1 "Interpretation for Freud and Heidegger: Parataxis and Disclosure," in the *International Review of Psycho-Analysis* (London) 9, 1982, pp. 67-74.

Contexts Mostly Personal

Following graduation in 1968, when I returned home from college to make up my mind about what to do next, it happened that I was close to Duquesne University, in Pittsburgh, Pennsylvania. Duquesne was one of only a few academic centers for the study of phenomenology and existentialism in the United States, the others being The New School for Social Research (now The New School University) and Fordham University, both in New York City. I eventually spent quite a lot of time at the New School library and completed my PhD at Fordham a few years after my lay psychoanalytic training. So prized were the Duquesne philosophy and psychology faculties that graduate students would drive to Pittsburgh from as far away as Cleveland, Ohio, to attend once-weekly evening classes in those departments. I enrolled at Duquesne in 1971 and took graduate courses in both departments.

My interest in philosophy only deepened, but I decided that my calling was therapy, a vocation that I saw was only enriched by reading in the areas of continental philosophy and existential psychology, which often overlapped. This was a stimulating time, especially since the philosophy program where I had been an undergraduate was solidly in the tradition of analytic philosophy, except for that one course and a pair of independent studies that I arranged on Sartre's *Being and Nothingness*. Until I went to Duquesne, then, I had been pretty much on my own as a reader in existential psychology and Continental philosophy.

While finishing my psychoanalytic training, I wrote a small book on Heidegger which I published with Philosophical Library in 1987. As for "doing" psychoanalysis and psychoanalytic psychotherapy, my aspirations for maintaining a free-standing practice as a therapist were challenged, however, since independent office practice was becoming less feasible, especially for lay psychoanalysts. Both of my analysts—medical and lay—had worked out of their homes and this is what I wanted to do. That became a challenging affair. More important, during the time I was accepting the changing practical situation, I experienced an intellectual turning point that had been on the horizon since 1965.

What was known somewhat ambiguously as existential psychotherapy had attracted my interest since college days. At Duquesne, it was taught by, among others, Jan van den Berg, the great Dutch phenomenological psychiatrist, whom I got to know. Oddly enough, however, I often found myself defending psychoanalysis in seminars on therapy. I should add that when I was an undergraduate student of psychology, Freud was still very much in fashion, but at that time I found his ideas to be incredulous. Then, twenty years later, they became gospel for me. But by the late 1990s, existential analysis again challenged my belief in the Freudian paradigm. The course I followed was a zig-zag between two pathways. One had been followed by Freud—the other was Heidegger's way.

Having finally fully acknowledged the influence of what I had read by Heidegger and psychiatrists influenced by him—Ludwig Binswanger, van den Berg, Laing, and Boss—my commitment to Freud's metapsychology dissolved. I was again incredulous about Freud, but now I understood why. Boss, I learned much later, had also experienced precisely the same change of heart during those very years.

I taught psychology and philosophy to undergraduates beginning in 1972 and thoroughly enjoyed all of them—the disciplines and the students. Among fellow faculty in the psychology department where I spent the last half of my teaching career (1994-2019), however, I was something of a puzzle. I was associated by my colleagues with both the Third Force in our field (humanistic psychology) and also the First Force (psychoanalysis). Both, they assured me, were hopelessly out of fashion. As a professor of psychology, my critique of the Second Force (behaviorism) was explicit from the start with students and colleagues alike. It had remained unchanged from the first time I read John B. Watson and B.F. Skinner.

In addition to abandoning classical psychoanalysis and its well-known modifications in favor of existential psychotherapy, I also came to realize that I had never been convinced by the underlying ideas of humanistic psychology as represented, for example, by Carl Rogers' person-centered (or client-centered) psychotherapy. In short, I could not see the human beings I worked with as either patients or clients. It took me a while to differentiate between the existential and humanistic approaches chiefly because they had not been sufficiently distinguished from each other by people claiming membership in one or the other group. This was because a shared critical stance toward psychoanalysis, cognitive-behavioral therapy, and psychopharmacology had led adherents of these two very different approaches to band together on certain occasions and issues, giving the general impression that they were, if not the same, very similar in inspiration and practice. In fact, they were not—not at all. Making that clear is yet another reason for returning to Boss.

There is one more personal context to consider and that is psychiatric practice itself. Without a degree in medicine, as I have said, I was not eligible for application to any clinical program anywhere in the United States that had the imprimatur of the International Psychoanalytic Association. Of course, Boss was welcomed with open arms by medical psychoanalysts in the early days of institute training because he was a doctor and a psychiatrist. Yes, there were a few non-medical psychoanalysts among Freud's first followers and Freud was not trained as a psychiatrist, but almost from the start the key for access to psychoanalytic training was the MD. A notable exception, of course, was Boss's almost exact contemporary, Erik Erikson (1902-1994).

My deep admiration for my first analyst and then mentor and friend never waned, but it turned out that he was unique among his colleagues in psychiatry and psychoanalysis. In my therapeutic relationship with him, I experienced what I imagine it must have been like to work with existential analysts such as R.D. Laing, van den Berg—and Boss. I realized this after I saw Laing in action in a video. Like Laing and Boss, he was also ambivalent about psychiatry. Was he, by any chance, humanistic? Not at all. He was an existential analyst. The bit of serendipity of our meeting was, I have decided, gods-given.

My point here is that all of these men were psychiatrists, but with a difference, especially since existential analysis and medical practice are incommensurable. They had access to the prescription pad and hospital privileges, but only occasionally made use of these adjunctives to therapy, especially when they had limited their time to private practice. None believed for a moment that what was called mental illness could be cured with chemicals. In some cases, certain drugs over the short term might prepare the way for therapy, but such substances were no substitute for what Pedro Laín Entralgo called "the therapy of the word." These men also understood that for short periods of time, life in the world of the regular routines that hospitalization provides might provide some individuals with respite from a chaotic environment, but its ultimate purpose was to pave the way for private therapy. None of them considered hospitalization to be genuinely therapeutic in itself. A few weeks in the mountains or on a cruise would do just as well. Laing was especially outspoken on this issue. For any existential analyst, the legal incarceration of a person in a hospital does and cannot be made to square with an emphasis on supporting a human being's fundamental existential freedom.

Here mention should be made of two other psychiatrists who have had a great deal of influence on me: Harry Stack Sullivan and Thomas Szasz. They, too, were outsiders of the first order but very different sorts of men. Sullivan, from rural upstate New York, and Szasz, an *emigré* from Hungary, were surely as stark contrasts in manner and style as one can imagine. I am not aware of audio or film records of Sullivan, in interview or at work. All I know is that he wrote badly but from all reports had remarkable therapeutic successes in a hospital setting considered by some to be magical. Szasz was masterful as a speaker and writer, but he was skeptical about the very concept of psychotherapy—period. In a way, Sullivan was perhaps even more controversial than Szasz (if that is possible). He managed to elude scrutiny by the psychiatric establishment while he worked. Szasz, on the other hand, cheerfully put himself on the firing line again and again among establishment psychiatrists. It is worth adding that Szasz had been in analysis with Therese Benedek, but Sullivan substituted an extended *Wanderjahr* for an equivalent number of years on the couch.

All this leads to an interesting question: Would Sullivan, Szasz, Laing, van den Berg, Boss, and my first analyst be welcome today among the ranks of psychiatrists? I doubt it. Having attended medical school, would they specialize in psychiatry in 2019? I doubt it. Nor, I believe, would individuals such as Sigmund Freud (who in any event was never especially interested in being a doctor and did not specialize in psychiatry), Carl Gustav Jung (a mystic at heart), and the rest have turned to therapy. The same might be said of non-medical therapists such as Rollo May and James Bugental, or my lay training analyst—and me. Boss, we know, originally thought he would be a painter. I have played the piano quite well since I was eight years old. And yet we did respond to a certain calling. Especially in our era of medicalization of everyday life, the dopamine hypothesis of psychological disorders, and campaigns by pharmaceutical houses directed at consumers to sell their doctors on the idea of prescribing certain medications for "my depression" or "my schizophrenia" (as scripts for certain television ads are now written for individuals to read), I think the people I have named would not be welcome in psychiatry. If they had gone to medical school, they might have become internists. As undergraduates, I doubt that any of them would have declared a major in psychology.

Given these contexts, mostly personal, I nevertheless remain committed to the idea of therapy, and in what follows I want to pose and pursue the question: Where is contemporary psychotherapy heading? I am convinced that therapy "works," but believe it cannot work and never has worked in the context of medical practice. Boss realized and accepted this at some level beginning in the mid-1940s, albeit ambivalently, and for that reason developed a psychoanalysis without the psyche as far as he could—what he finally let be known in English as "da-seinanalysis."[1]

In time, I hope to take a look at the other individuals named above—especially Jan van den Berg and R.D. Laing—with a view to understanding the part they played in the modern history of the therapy of the word. I begin with Medard Boss, however, because of his unique association with the foundational thinker of existential analysis, Martin Heidegger, who in every case (except Sullivan, to the best of my knowledge) was the acknowledged source for these psych-

---

1   This was Boss's final approved English version of the German term *Daseinsanalyse* as it appears in his preface to the "American translation" of the Zollikon seminars, which he edited for publication during the last months of his life. Perhaps it was less than helpful in conveying his ideas. For that reason, I have chosen to speak from here on out of his *existential analysis*. In the following section, I will look closely at terminological difficulties introduced by a variety of translational *faux pas* of this and related German words, knowing that my audience will for the most part be students of Boss and psychotherapy who are limited to English translations of his works and related texts. My own translation decisions are in play in the next section and might prove helpful when retranslations are made of Boss's papers and books.

iatrists of ideas that challenged medicine as the appropriate home for those who want to provide therapy for other human beings. Boss is the person with whom to begin because of his unique background, which includes a little-known crisis as a human being that nonetheless could not bring him to officially break with his past as a medical man. In any event, it seems obvious to me that the story of therapy—the most human of callings—must be a story about particular human beings as much as about their ideas.

My goal is to spark a renaissance of interest in that period of time between the heyday of psychoanalysis and the beginning of the pharmacracy by looking at the work of Medard Boss and what it may yet have to contribute to salvaging therapy from psychiatry. But in Boss's case, is this a realistic goal? Interest can result only from the availability of material to read and become interested in. As we know, this is limited, but the problem can be remedied.

Introduction

The time has come to revisit the contribution of Medard Boss to therapy. Why? There are several reasons. For scholars, the most important is the recent publication of Martin Heidegger's notes for the Zollikon seminars. The notes, gathered from Heidegger's *Nachlaß*, must now be taken into consideration in a re-evaluation of Boss's publication in 1987 of the protocols of those thirteen fabled sessions for psychiatrists and others (1959-1969), supplemented by Boss's notes from private conversations (or dialogues) with Heidegger (1961-1972), and excerpts from some of Heidegger's letters to Boss (1947-1971).

A second reason for returning to Boss's work is to introduce a new generation of prospective therapists to his singular perspective and its potential for taking a fresh perspective on therapy in an era when psychopharmacology and cognitive behavior modification are becoming more and more suspect. Boss, I believe, is our best way out of the medical model by which psychiatry and clinical psychology have been bewitched since the first generation of psychoanalysts, working for the most part in Berlin and London, limited prospective newcomers to psychoanalysis to men and women who were medical doctors. Boss, who experienced this period first-hand, nonetheless came closest among the early generations of psychoanalysts to make a turn in the direction of a genuinely human therapy. Why he was ultimately unable to do so will become clear. So also will what can be done to fully realize the tendency he envisioned.

Introduction

From Ludwig Binswanger, via Boss, to Alice Holzhey-Kunz, *Daseinsanalyse* has been correctly understood as a form of psychoanalysis.[1] We must never forget this. What it means is that, like psychoanalysis, existential analysis as Boss left it for us remained grounded in the medical model, which is marked by *interventional looking after* another human being, what Heidegger termed *einspringende Fürsorge*. Like a parent, the psychoanalyst steps in and takes over, no matter how passive he may appear to be as a listener suspended in free-floating attention. Concern of this kind, however, inevitably dispossesses the other of his freedom.

One of Freud's analysands for a brief period of time, Boss blazed a trail he himself could not follow to its destination; namely, a kind of psychotherapy without the psyche that came to be known as *Daseinsanalyse*. A genuine therapy, Boss saw, had to be based on a view of the human being that does not begin with the assumption of an object of some sort, such as the psyche or ego, secreted away in a hypothetical physical or mental apparatus in a human being. The therapy he envisioned is oriented to existence, not to an ego, subject, self, or psyche. Its means is *way-making looking after*, what Heidegger termed *vorausspringende Fürsorge*. This fundamental distinction between two kinds of concern has been forgotten in the often Byzantine discussions of the great variety of approaches generally term existential, but it is essential to everything that follows.[2] That Boss also understood the psyche as man's *soul* as Freud did remained as problematic for him. We will return to this.

There is another dimension of Boss's approach to therapy to keep in mind and that is his "Indian experience." He compared ideas learned

---

1 See as bookends Ludwig Binswanger [1930-1957], *Being-in-the-World. Selected Papers* (New York: Basic Books, 1963) ["Dream and Existence" (1930), "Freud's Conception of Man in the Light of Anthropology (1936), "Freud and the Magna Carta of Clinical Psychiatry" (1936), "Heidegger's Analytic of Existence and Its Meaning for Psychiatry" (1949), "The Case of Lola Voss" (1949), "Extravagance" (1949), and "Introduction" to *Schizophrenia* (1957)] and Alice Holzhey-Kunz, *Daseinsanalysis* (London: Free Association Books, 2014).
2 This distinction is made by Heidegger in *Sein und Zeit* (1927), GA 2 (11977), ¶ 26. On the vagaries of existential therapies see, for example, the recently published *Wiley World Handbook of Existential Therapy* (Chichester: John Wiley and Sons Ltd., 2019).

Introduction

at the feet of several spiritual leaders in India to what he had heard from Heidegger in the Black Forest of Southwest Germany and found remarkable similarities. He also saw a likeness between spiritual growth in the Eastern tradition with aspects of the self-illumination of one who meets with a genuine therapist in the setting of existential analysis.

What follows now is an attempt to trace the origins of existential analysis in psychoanalysis and follow the leads Boss provided to describe how a genuine *therapeut* might practice.[1]

First, however, I will pause to consider in general some of the problems of terminology and translation using a recent document in which *Daseinsanalyse* is discussed by two leading European existential psychotherapists.

---

1 The German noun *Therapeut* is currently used for our English word 'psychotherapist.' I have come to prefer the English transliteration *therapeut* to the word therapist, not to copy the German word but in reference to the original *Therapeutes* or *Therapeutae*, members of an ascetic Essene sect that lived during the first century of the Common Era. See my two-part essay, "The Return of the Therapeut," in *The International Journal of Psychotherapy* 18(1), March 2014, pp. 5-18, and 18(2), July 2014, pp. 5-20.

Problems of Terminology and Translation

Boss is synonymous with *Daseinsanalyse* (existential analysis), yet confusion about the word and the modality of psychotherapy it denotes has existed since the word first appeared in the literature of psychology and psychiatry in the work of Ludwig Binswanger. Confusions led to misunderstandings among both well-wishers and critics of Boss.

A recent exchange between contemporaries, one a lay analyst and student of Boss, Alice Holzhey-Kunz, and her colleague among existential therapists, the medical doctor and protegé of Viktor Frankl, Alfried Längle, illustrates difficulties that persist even today among German-speaking existential therapists in being clear about just what existence means.[1] The dialogue between two of the most eminent existential therapists illustrates the complicated linguistic setting which the present study addresses. It is also important because it contrasts existential analysis with other modalities in the tradition of existential psychotherapy.

The passages provide me with an opportunity to suggest what I think are clear translations of key terms (**bolded**) that will be used through-

---

1 Alfried Längle and Alice Holzhey-Kunz, *Existenzanalyse und Daseinsanalyse* (Vienna: Facultas, 2008). See also a even very recent dialogue between Holzhey-Kunz and the physician and *Daseinsanalytiker* (existential analyst) Tamás Fazekas, "Daseinsanalysis. A Dialogue," in *Existential Therapy. Legacy, Vibrancy, and Dialogue* (London: Routledge, 2012), pp. 35-51. The ongoing uneasy relation between medical and lay practice is not acknowledged, but it is an evident undertone of the exchange.

out this study. These are summarized in the Glossary. For each passage the German text is provided in a footnote.

Alfried Längle (AL): At the heart of **analysis of existing** (ES) is the concept of "**existing**." By this is understood meaningful living in the world informed by freedom and responsibility.... / The understanding of **existing** of ES is in the tradition of **philosophy of existing** (e.g., [Søren] Kierkegaard [1813-1855], 1844 [*Begrebet Angest* [*The Concept of Anxiety*]]; [Martin] Heidegger [1889-1976], 1927 [*Sein und* Zeit [*Being and Time*]]; [Karl] Jaspers [1883-1969],1938 [*Existenzphilosophie* [*Philosophy of Existing*], 1948 [*Der philosophische Glaube* [*Philosophical Belief*]]; Jean-Paul Sartre [1905-1980], 1943 [*L'être et le* néant [*Being and Nothingness*]]; [Otto Friedrich] Bollnow [1903-1991], 1943 [*Existenzphilosophie* [*Philosophy of Existing*]]; [Max] Müller [1906-1994], 1949 [*Existenzphilosophie im geistige Leben der* Gegenwart [*Philosophy of Existing in the Spiritual Life of the Present*]]; [Hannah] Arendt [1906-1975], 1990 [*Was ist Existenzphilosophie?* [*What Is Philosophy of Existing?*]]; [Franz] Zimmermann [b. 1941], 1977 [[*Einführung in die Existenzphilosophie* [*Introduction to Philosophy of Existing*]; [Nolberto] Espinosa [1929-2014], 1998 ["On the Task of Logotherapy and **Analysis of Existing** in the Postmetaphysical Era," in *Existenzanalyse* **15**(3), 4-12]). Man sees himself as embedded in a world. **Existence** is being-in-the-world, as Heidegger puts it (see Holzhey-Kunz 203 f. [present volume].... That which the person perceives as 'his own' is not only the internalization of external experience, but rather always has a genuine, unmistakable origin in the person himself (pp. 23-24).[1]

---

1 Im Mittelpunkt der Existenzanalyse (ES) steht der Begriff "Existenz." Darunter wird ein *sinvolles, in Freiheit und Verantwortung* gestaltetes Leben in der Welt verstanden.... / Das Existenzverständnis der EA steht in der Tradition der Existenzphilosophie (z.B. Kierkegaard 1848; Heidegger 1979; Jaspers 1956a, 1974; Sartre 1946; Bollnow 1965; Müller 1964; Arendt 1990; Zimmermann 1992; Espinosa 1998). In ihm wird der Mensch als eingebettet in einer Welt gesehen. Das Dasein ist 'In-der-Welt-Sein,' wie es Heidegger formuliert (vgl. Holzhey-Kunz 203 f.).... Das, was die Person als 'das Eigene' empfindet, ist nicht nur Internalisierung von äußeren Erfahrung, sondern hat immer auch einen genuinen, unverwechselbaren Ursprung in der Person selbst.

Problems of Terminology and Translation

A central idea of **existentialist** psychotherapy runs: Man "is" not, he "**ek-sists.**" The central concept "**to ek-sist**" means that man is not set (determined) in his essence. Instead, he is essentially oriented to [the] world, "extraverted (cf. [Max] Scheler [1874-1928], 1928 [*Die Stellung des Menschen im Kosmos* (*The Place of Man in the Cosmos*)] and carries out his **existing** in a dialogically encountering indissoluble interwovenness with the "others" of the world (p. 80).[1]

Existential analysis, analysis of existing but also Gestalt therapy and process-oriented talk therapy (Hans Swildens [b. 1924) can count as **existentialist** psychotherapy:

> **Existentialist** orientations can be found not only in explicit representatives of **existentialist** thinking such as [Medard] Boss [1903-1990], [Ludwig] Binswanger [1881-1966], [Wolfgang] Blankenburg [1928-2002], [James] Bugental [1915-2008], [Gion] Condrau [1919-2006], [Viktor] Frankl [1905-1997], [Alfried] Längle [b. 1951], [Rollo] May, but also in **analytic** approaches (e.g., individual psychology [Alfred Adler] [1870-1937] and analytical psychology, such as [Igor] Caruso [1914-1981], [Carl Gustav] Jung [1875-1961] and in addition [Henri] Ey [1900-1977], [Viktor] von Gebsattel [1883-1976], [Eugène] Minkowski [1885-1972], [Erwin] Straus [1891-1975]), and in humanistically oriented neo-analytic (e.g., [Otto] Rank [1884-1939], [Karen] Horney [1885-1952], [Erich] Fromm [1900-1980]) and the more fundamental personality-based [approaches] of humanistic psychology (e.g., [Abraham] Maslow [1908-1970], [Fritz] Perls [1893-1970], [Carl] Rogers [1902-1987]) (Stumm & Längle 2000, 180) (p. 81).[2]

---

1 Ein zentraler Gedanke der existentiellen Psychotherapie besagt: Der Mensch "ist" nicht, er "existiert." Der zentral Begriff "existieren" bedeutet, dass der Mensch in seinem Wesen nicht festgelegt (determiniert) ist. Er ist vielmehr wesenhalt ausgerichtet auf Welt, ist "weltoffen" (vgl. Scheler 1978) und vollzieht seine Existenz in einem dialogisch-beggegnenden, und aufhebbaren Verwobensein mit dem "anderem" der Welt.

2 Als existentielle Psychotherapie könne die Daseinsanalyse, die Existenzanalyse, aber auch die Gestalttherapie und die Prozessorientierte Gesprächspsychotherapie (nach Hans Swildens) gelten:

Problems of Terminology and Translation

Analysis of existing and **analysis of existence** are two classic European approaches in therapy that are based on a long significant intellectual tradition: **philosophy of existing** and phenomenology. On their foundations, in the thirties and forties of the last century logotherapy and **analysis of existing** emerged in Austria and, in Switzerland, **analysis of existence**. The founders were, on the one hand, Viktor Frankl (1905-1997), and on the other, Ludwig Binswanger (1881-1966) and Medard Boss (1903-1990) (p. 13).[1]

'**Existing**' and '**existence**' are related terms, and both approaches also speak of themselves as '**analysis**' (p. 13).[2]

Viktor Frankl, the founder of **analysis of existing**, saw searching for meaning as central to his approach to psychotherapy. Man does not merely want to satisfy needs; he primarily wants to *understand* what

---

> Existentielle Orientierungen lassen sich aber nicht nur bei expliziten Vertretern des existentiellen Denkens wie Boss, Binswanger, Blankenburg, Bugental, Condrau, Frankl, Längle, May, Tellenbach, Yalom finden, sondern auch bei analytischen Richtungen (z.B. Individualpsychologie und Analytische Psychologie nach Caruso, Jung, weiters bei Ey, v. Gebsattel, Minkowsky [sic], Straus) und humanistisch ausgerichteten Neo-Analytikern (z.B. Rank, Horney, Fromm) und Gründerpersönlichkeiten der Humanistischen Psychologie (z.B. Maslow, Perls, Rogers (Stumm & Längle 2000, 180).
> [The reference is to "Existentielle Psychotherapie," in Gerhard Stumm and Alfred Pritz (eds,), *Wörterbuch der Psychotherapie* (Vienna: Springer, 2000), pp. 180-181. Längle's use of *analytisch* in reference to Adler, Jung and others and neo-analysts refer to psychoanalysis and are shorthand for it. That Jung's modality came to be known as Analytic Psychology adds a further element of possible confusion.]

1 Existenzanalyse und Daseinsanalyse sind zwei klassische europäische Therapierichtungen, die auf einer langen bedeutsam Geistestradition beruhen: der Existenzphilosophie und der Phänomenologie. Auf ihren Grundlagen entstanden in der Dreißiger- und Vierzigerjahren des letzten Jahrhunderts in Österreich die *Logotherpie und Existenzanalyse*, in der Schweiz die *Daseinsanalyse*. Begründer waren Viktor Frankl (1905-1997) einerseits, Ludwig Binswanger (1881-1966) und Medard Boss (1903-1990) anderseits.
2 'Existenz' und 'Dasein' sind verwandte Begriffe, und beide Richtungen nennen sich darüber auch noch 'Analyse'. [Here Längle refers to the second element in the two forms of existential therapy being discussed, which he considers to be based on psychoanalysis and a procedure of taking apart or dissecting.]

Problems of Terminology and Translation

he lives *for* and can endure suffering if he has a '*wherefore*'. Frankl therefore spoke more about 'logotherapy', where 'logos' denotes 'meaning'. Logotherapy was for him a complement to conventional psychotherapy, which of course in the 1920s and 1930s referred only to Freud and Adler (p. 14).[1]

We see the question of meaning as [an] **existentialist** question, and thus also as [the] 'primary question', which is often relatively clear in everyday life, but can sometimes feel urgent. To ask about *meaning* in the **analysis of existing** and logotherapy is to search for something of personal value to me—an action, an experience, an enduring.... What is 'special' about **analysis of existing** I would see in the fact that it takes seriously the central anthropological understanding of human freedom and that it offers assistance in order to live with determination (pp. 14-15).[2]

...

Alice Holzhey-Kunz (AH-K): The concept "**existing**" is already common in philosophy before Heidegger and it is used to indicate that something actually occurs, that it **is really there**, and that it is not just a figment of the imagination. Its counter-concept is "essence," which stands for what constitutes the nature of a thing or a human being....

---

1   Viktor Frankl, der Begründer der Existenzanalyse, sah ihm Einziehen der Sinnsuche des Menschen in die Psychotherapie das Zentrale seiner Richtung. Der Mensch will nicht einfach Bedürfnisse befriedigen, er will in erster Linie *verstehen, wofür* er lebt, und kann ein Leiden nur ertragen, wenn er ein '*Wozu*' hat. Frankl sprach darum mehr von der 'Logotherapie'—wobei 'Logos' so viel wie 'Sinn' bedeutet. Logotherapie war für ihn eine 'Ergänzung' der herkömmlichen Psychotherapie', was sich in den 1920er- und 1930er-Jahren natürlich nur auf Freud und Adler bezog.

2   Wir sehen die Sinnfrage als *existenzielle Frage* und somit auch also 'Urfrage', die im Alltag oft relative klar ist, aber manchmal sehr unter den Fingern brennen kann. Nach *Sinn* zu fragen, heißt in der Existenzanalyse und Logotherapie, nach dem *fühlbaren Wert* zu suchen, den etwas—eine Handlung, ein Erleben, ein Erleiden—für mich persönlich hat.... Die 'Eigene' der Existenzanalyse würde ich darin sehen, dass sie Ernst macht mit dem zentral anthropologische Verständnis der *Freiheit* des Menschen und dass sie Hilfestellung anbietet, um mit *Entschiedenheit* zu leben.

Problems of Terminology and Translation

Heidegger goes against this tradition of thought about the being of man when he provocatively declares: "The nature of **existence** is in its **existing**" (SZ 42). This sentence is so unheard of [i.e., surprising] that it has largely remained unheard [i.e., acknowledged]. Its meaning can be understood only if one recognizes that Heidegger uses the old concept of "**existing**" but gives it an entirely different meaning. / In a critical transformation of ancient ontology the [Heidegger's] essential argument consists in limiting talk of **existing** and **[what it is] to exist** to humanity. The word '**existing**' is used exclusively for the description of being *human*. But, in contrast to [things] being extant and occurring, the human being just **ek-sists**. Things or living beings are extant or even—like tools crafted by man—available, but they have no **existing** [about them], while man is never only extant or available, but is precisely **[to] "ek-sist."** The special thing about **existing** in comparison to merely being extant is that only man **is** not *simpliciter*, but has "**to be**": "The essence of this **being** [i.e., of existence] is in its **to-being**" (SZ 42). For Heidegger, therefore, the special character of man is "**to-being,**" which fundamentally differentiates him not only from inanimate things but also from non-human living things (p. 201).[1]

---

1 Der Begriff "Existenz" ist schon vor Heidegger in der Philosophie gebräuchlich und wird verwendet, um so sage, dass etwas tatsächlich vorkommt, dass es realiter existiert und nicht nur rein Hirngespinst darstellt. Sein Gegenbegriff ist "Essenz," der für das steht, was eine Sache oder einem Menschen in seinem Wesen ausmacht. ... Gegen diese Denktradition geht Heidegger bei der Bestimmung des Menschseins an, indem er provokativ erklärt: "*Das Wesen des Daseins liegt in seiner Existenz*" (SZ 42). Dieser Satz ist so unerhört, dass er auch mithin ungehört geblieben ist. Seine Bedeutung lässt sich nur verstehen, wenn man erkennt, dass Heidegger zwar den altern Begriff "Existenz" verwendet, ihm aber einen ganz anderen Sinn gibt. / Der wesentliche Stritt in der kritischen Transformation der alten Ontologie besteht darin, die Rede von Existenz und Existieren auf Menschen zu beschränken. Das Wort 'Existenz' dient fortan ausschließlich der Beschriebung *menschlichen* Seins: Nur der Mensch "existiert" steht im Gegensatz zu "Vorhandenheit" oder "Vorkommen." Dinge oder Lebewesen sind vorhanden oder auch—wie die von Menschen geschaffen Werkzeuge—zuhanden, aber sie habe keine Existenz, während der Mensch niemals nur vorhanden oder zuhanden ist, sondern eben "existiert." Das Besondere des Existierens gegenüber dem bloßen Vorhandensein liegt darin, dass nur der Mensch nicht einfach ist, sondern "zu sein" hat: "*Das Wesen dieses Seienden* [d.h. *des Menschen*] *liegt in seinem Zu-sein*" (SZ 42). Im "Zu-sein" liegt also für Heidegger das Besondere des Menschen, das ihn nicht nur von den leblosen Dingen, sondern auch von den nichtmenschlichen Lebewesen grundlegend unterscheidet.

Problems of Terminology and Translation

I would like to begin with Freud. What is 'special' about **analysis of existence** can be formulated only in relation to psychoanalysis. Somewhat exaggerated, one could say that **analysis of existence** is the product of thinking together Freud and Heidegger (plus Sartre). **Analysis of existence** takes up Freud's discoveries and places them in the context of the basic **existential** [in the Sartrean existentialist tradition] situation of man. This is because we humans are not simply subject (like all living things) to unalterable conditions of being but also secretly *know* about them, so that our lifestyle is always determined by knowing about the *conditio humana*, even if we do not expressly consider it (p. 14).[1]

How can you put the main focus on the positive in **analysis of existing** when you are based on the **philosophy of existing**? We know this elsewhere in the inborn striving for self-actualization of the humanistic psychology of Carl Rogers (p. 17).[2]

This exchange between two preeminent representatives of existential psychotherapy spotlights the principal problematic term in our discussion of Boss: existence. The discussion is essentially about the difference between the concepts of existing [*Existenz*] and existence [*Dasein*]. There are problems, however.

Dr. Längle, for his part, conflates existence and existing, glossing existing with Heidegger's existence as ek-sisting or standing out into the world. He also lumps together analysis of existing (and logo-

---

1 Bei Freud möchte ich gerne anknüpfen. Das 'Eigene' der Daseinsanalyse kann man nur in Bezug auf die Psychoanalyse formulieren. Etwas überspitzt könnte man sagen, dass die Daseinsanalyse das Produkt eines Zusammendenkens von Freud und Heidegger (plus Sartre) ist. Die Daseinsanalyse nimmt die Entdeckungen Freuds auf und stellt sie in der Zusammenhang der existentiellen Grundsituation des Menschen. Diese besteht darin, dass wir Menschen nicht einfach (wie alles Lebendige) unabänderlichen Seinsbedingungen unterworfen sind, sondern dass wir um diese insgeheim auch *wissen*, so das unsere Lebensführung immer von diesem Wissen um die *conditio humana* mitbestimmt ist, auch wenn wir gar nicht ausdrücklich darüber nachdenken.
2 Warum könnt ihr in der Existenzanalyse einen so positiven Schwerpunkt legen, wo ihr doch auf dem Boden der Existenzphilosophie steht? Das kennen wir sonst vom angeborenen Selbstrealisierungsstreben in der Humanistischen Psychologie von Carl Rogers.

therapy) with existential analysis as forms of *existentialist* psychotherapy, which, he claims, includes representatives as diverse as Boss and Carl Rogers. His context is philosophy of existing *and phenomenology*, which together, he says, are the common source of both his analysis of existing and existential analysis.

According to Längle, philosophy of existing begins with Kierkegaard and includes Heidegger and Sartre as well as Jaspers, with whom the philosophy is usually associated. From early on, of course, Heidegger explicitly distanced himself from Jaspers' philosophy, and Längle certainly knew this. He focuses on the term 'analysis' in analysis of existing and existential analysis, but as we will see, an analysis (Freud) and an analytics (Heidegger) are quite different matters, and the latter is in the background of existential analysis. These imprecisions are unfortunate and confusing. So is Längle's claim that Frankl was the founder of analysis of existing as well as logotherapy. Indeed, Längle often speaks of the two interchangeably, which allows him to see both analysis of existing and logotherapy as focused on "searching for meaning" and making possible "meaningful living." Like Binswanger's, his approach is anthropological, but Heidegger, who is cited as a source for analysis of existing, was careful to distinguish his analytics of existence from anthropology, as well as from psychology and biology.[1]

In her contribution, Holzhey-Kunz always has in mind existence, not existing, yet what stands out in her part of the dialogue is a comment on existing, the central term in Längle's analysis of existing. She first quotes what is perhaps the most famous sentence from Heidegger's *Sein und Zeit*: "The nature of existence is in its existing." A few lines later, she then quotes a sentence that *precedes* this one in Heidegger's section in his book on "The Theme of the Analytics of Existence," but in glossing the word *Seiende* (an instance of what is there) in reference to *Dasein*, she mistakenly interpolates "[that is, man [*Mensch*]]."

But Heidegger was not writing from an anthropological perspective about humanity or a given man or woman, but rather about existence [*Dasein*], the essence of which, he says in the earlier sentence, "is

---

1 GA 2, 60.

in its to-being [*Zu-sein*]." In both places he is writing about existence, not humanity. Holzhey-Kunz is therefore not accurate in inferring that for Heidegger "the special character of man is 'to-being' [or to-ness], which fundamentally differentiates him not only from inanimate things but also from non-human living things." That is precisely the special character of existence. In an effort to distinguish human beings from all other sorts of beings, which Heidegger does, Holzhey-Kunz has made an error in equating existence with humanity. Since this is such an important matter in making clear Boss's unique grounding in Heidegger, a few more words are in order.

Heidegger's great value was to have dug beneath the foundations of Western ontology as metaphysics, which had been concerned with human beings as beings just like every other being found in nature. Instead, he proposed a study of the grounding phenomenon for the very possibility of ontology, namely, the questioner asking about what is there and carrying out an activity that is the origin of philosophizing, which yields an ontology. In his study he took up the task of (what was perhaps not well named) fundamental ontology, since as seemingly a kind of ontology, it is easily confused with the division of Western philosophy that since Wolff and Baumgartner we have known as ontology as distinguished from logic, metaphysics, epistemology, ethics, and aesthetics.

Heidegger's dismantling of metaphysics was to have been about exposing the arbitrariness of this taxonomy. He nevertheless chose to use the compound *Fundamentalontologie*. His use of the term *vorontologisch* (pre-ontological) is helpful in conceptually placing existence ahead of humanity as the topic of his fundamental-ontological analytics. The important point is that Heidegger did not undertake an anthropology or science of man, as Längle mistakenly believed, but rather a description of the "categories" unique to existence [*Dasein*] as ek-sisting [*Existieren*]—the existentatives [*Existentiale*]. As his well-known exchange with Jean Beaufret made very clear, he was not concerned in *Sein und Zeit* with humanity, but instead with an analytics of existence.[1]

---

1 "Brief über den 'Humanismus,'" in *Wegmarken* (1967), *GA* 9 (1976), pp. 313-364.

Problems of Terminology and Translation

The confounding term in Heidegger's vocabulary, then, is not *Dasein* but *Existenz*. This is evident in the exchange we are reviewing here. I suspect he spent many hours regretting having written that second sentence early on in *Sein und Zeit* and not having left things well enough alone in saying that the essence of existence is its to-being or to-ness.[1]

In the last passage quoted, Holzhey-Kunz shows herself to be closer to Längle than one might have anticipated and to that precise extent at a distance from Heidegger, whose analytics of existence was the core of her mentor's revision of psychoanalysis and psychotherapy. Like Längle, she includes Sartre among the sources of her own version of analysis of existence. Holzhey-Kunz's existential analysis is in some respects an existentialist interpretation of psychoanalysis and might be compared to Sartre's *psychanalyse existentielle*, which is, however, neither Freudian psychoanalysis (or a revision of it such as object relations theory or self psychology) nor existential analysis.

---

1   Taken together, the two sentences quoted by Holzhey-Kunz allow us to conclude that, for Heidegger, the essence of existence is in its existing [*Existenz*], that is to say (and better said), its to-ness or to-being [*Zu-sein*]. Marginal notes available since the 1977 *Complete Edition* version of *Sein und Zeit* would have been known to Holzhey-Kunz (and Boss) but they are not mentioned here. For example, in a note to "Zu-sein" in the first of those two memorable sentences quoted, he wrote: "*daß is zu seyn 'hat'; Bestimmung!*" (GA 2, 55, note d)—"that it 'has' to *be*; [this is its] determination!" The verb in its old spelling points to Heidegger's understanding of the usage of the verb as transitive, not in usual intransitive sense where "to be" requires an objective complement. The latter usage of the verb is a feature of metaphysical thinking, which misses the power of the verb. Earlier in *Sein und Zeit*, Heidegger had referred to *Existenz* as the "Sein des Menschen" (GA 2, 16, note a)—"the [to] be of man." This is not the place for a longer commentary on Heidegger, but for whatever reasons of misunderstanding or incomplete understanding, it is a basic mistake to equate existence [*Dasein*] and existing [*Existenz*], which is the "[to] be of man." This error seems to have persisted in much of the thinking about existential analysis [*Daseinsanalysis*], however. Another distinction, familiar to those who have studied Heidegger, may make this plainer. Existence is an ontological matter while existing is ontic. And so it happens: "Die Frage der Existenz ist eine ontische 'Angelegenheit' des Daseins" (GA 2, 17).—"The question about existing is an ontic 'cause' for existence." In the end, *Existenz* is a *who*, not a *what* (an entity of whatever sort). But here is the crux of the matter: *Dasein* is neither ontic nor ontological and in this lies its singularity. Existence is neither a what nor a who. Given what is there (*das Seiende*), existence is fundamental for making the distinction between the two.

Problems of Terminology and Translation

Holzey-Kunz is nonetheless correct in observing that to understand analysis of existence one must begin with Freud's analysis of the soul. This was also Boss's starting point but his ambivalence about psychoanalysis would preoccupy him throughout his encounter with Heidegger, even in its early stages.[1]

---

[1] We know that Heidegger only reluctantly and under pressure from Boss read Freud. His principal interest was in Freud's observations about therapy, not the metapsychology. Again ironically, however, his hope was that speaking to Boss's colleagues in psychiatry might have a favorable effect on their work as medical doctors, even as it became clear to Boss that existential analysis could not be a form of medical practice.

Part I
"Da-seinanalysis" in Print

The preceding dialogue from 2008 is still current in demonstrating confusions that plague practitioners about what counts as existential analysis and how to understand it. The participants in the dialogue had the benefit of reading Boss in the original German. One of them, Holzhey-Kunz, was Boss's student and colleague. But what of those who have relied on English translations of his work? What is unclear to our interlocutors remains unclear in most cases to the present generation of existential psychotherapists, including existential analysts.

In order to understand the situation that such individuals face in appreciating Boss's contribution, I now turn to his book-length publications and their translations in which his existential analysis was formulated. All of them reflect the influence of Martin Heidegger's thought on his work as a therapist and reflect the refinement of an existential analysis that Heidegger sanctioned. They culminate in his *Grudriß der Medizin* (1971) which is the fruit of the Zollikon seminars (1959-1969).

A. Early Publications Influenced by Martin Heidegger

Boss was influenced by Heidegger at least as early as his book on sexual perversions (paraphilias). Earlier publications do not hint at the effect of Heidegger's thought on Boss's development as a psychotherapist.

1. *Meaning and Content of Sexual Perversions.*

A Daseinsanalytic Contribution to the Psychopathology of the Phenomenon of Love is a study of the paraphilic disorders or, as they were called in Medard Boss's time, the sexual perversions. As the subtitle says, however, it is also a study of love [*Liebe*] or intimacy.[1] The subtitle

---

1 *Sinn und Gehalt der sexuellen Perversionen. Ein daseinsanalytischer Beitrag zur Psychopathologie des Phänomens der Liebe* (Bern: Huber, 1947 [= SG1]; 2nd ("English language") ed., New York: Grune & Stratton, 1949 [= MC]; 2nd revised and expanded ed., 1952 [= SG2]; 3rd further revised and expanded ed., Munich: Kindler, 1966 [= SG3]; 4th ed., Frankfurt: Fischer, 1984, 2017. *Meaning and Content of Sexual Perversions. A Daseinsanalytic Contribution to the Psychopathology of the Phenomenon of Love* is the translation made by Liese Lewis Abell, PhD, a psychologist at Goldwater Memorial Hospital (City Hospital) on Welfare Island (now Roosevelt Island), then a massive facility for New York City's indigent chronically ill. Her only other scholarly work seems to have been a journal article on biochemistry published in *The American Heart Journal*.

A. Early Publications Influenced by Martin Heidegger

also makes clear that it is a book influenced by Martin Heidegger's analytics [*Analytik*][1] of existence [*Dasein*].

---

1 Much misunderstanding by psychologists and psychiatrists has resulted from confusing Heidegger's use of the nouns *Analytik* and *Analyse* in *Sein und Zeit*. Heidegger uses both words in the course of developing his fundamental ontology. Boss is referring to the *Analytik* (analytics) of existence [Dasein]. The word *Analytik* is Heidegger's neologism. It does not appear in Grimm or even in many standard popular German dictionaries. *Analyse* is a common noun that converts nicely to *analysis* (from the Greek word referring to the "breaking apart" of something into is constituents, as in a chemical analysis), but *Analytik* speaks to something else. It is, I believe, an allusion to Aristotle's analytics (prior and posterior), two treatises on logic belonging to his organon. I believe Heidegger had this context in mind when he coined the term *Analytik* and we should understand his *Daseinsanalytik* in terms of it. He was not thinking of chemical analysis. We should bear in mind that Freud's *Psycho-Analyse* was still a novelty when he wrote *Sein und* Zeit in the mid-1920s. In *Sein und Zeit* in addition to an analytics of existence [*Analytik des Daseins*], we often find terms such as ontological analytics [*ontologische Analytik*], existentive analytics [*existenziale Analytik*], and existentive-temporal analytics [*existenzial-zeitliche Analytik*]. In two places, however, he writes about something else, namely, an analytics of existing [*Analytik der Existenz*]. The formulation "*thematic* analytics of existing [thematische *Analytik der Existenz*]" is somehow out of character with the analytics of existence. It is found only in the Introduction (§7) of *Sein und Zeit* and in (§83), the book's concluding section, where Heidegger quotes his own definition of philosophy presented in the introduction. But he also speaks of analysis [*Analyse*] in the conventional sense. For example, Heidegger heads the first chapter of the first division of Part One of his book "The Exposition of the Task of a Preparatory Existential Analysis," which begins with §9, "The Theme of the Analytics of Existence." He writes of a fundamental analysis [*Fundamentalanalyse*] of existence as well as "The Delimitation of the Existentive Analysis of Death from Other Interpretations of the Phenomenon" and "The Temporality of Existence and the Tasks Arising from It on Repeating the Existentive Analysis." Is there a confusion here? When Heidegger speaks of an *Analytik*, it is, with the two exceptions mentioned, always in connection with the structure [*Struktur*] of *Dasein*. In sum: The goal of his analytics is the discernment of the *logos* (meaning) of existence and that is the ultimate purpose of his fundamental ontology; on the other hand, when he writes of the "task of a preparatory analysis of *Dasein*," he has in mind the conventional sense of a procedure that dissects or takes something apart, takes it to pieces. Finally, in the crucial expression "analytics of existing [*Existenz*]," however, we find something unique in Heidegger's masterwork, and it is precisely in the two passages where he defines philosophy: "Philosophie ist universale phänomenologische Ontologie, ausgehend von der Hermeneutik des Daseins, die als *Analytik der Existenz* das Ende des Leitfadens alles philosophischen Fragens dort festgemacht hat, woraus es *entspringt* und wohin es *zurückschlägt*:

A. Early Publications Influenced by Martin Heidegger

The book deserves our careful consideration, since in its three editions (1947, 1952, 1966) it is a record of powerful influence of Heidegger's thought on Boss's work as a psychiatrist and psychoanalyst over a period of two decades, including between the second and third editions his experience in the Zollikon seminars.

The first edition of *Meaning and Content of Sexual Perversions* already reflects Boss's disenchantment with psychoanalysis, but the existential analysis that he developed was nonetheless a modification of psychoanalysis. The name *Daseinsanalyse* originated with Ludwig Binswanger's application to psychiatry of Heidegger, as he understood the thinker's analytics of existence. Boss had good reason to make use of the term, since it was Binswanger who had introduced him to Heidegger's book and the two men worked together at the Kreuzlingen Sanatorium, located about 45 miles from Zürich on Lake Constance (the Bodensee), which Binswanger directed. Binswanger was evidently the first psychiatrist to introduce Heidegger to the medical establishment.

"Philosophy is universal phenomenological ontology, starting out from the hermeneutics of existence, which as the *analytics of existing* [emphasis added] has fixed the end of the guiding line for all philosophical questioning, from where it arises [*entspringt*] and to which it *returns* [Heidegger's emphasis]." A marginal note to the word *Existenz* in (§7) is reproduced in the *Complete Edition* version of the work: "'Existenz' fundamentalontologisch, d. h. auf Wahrheit des Seins selber bezogen, und nur so!": "'Existing' fundamental-ontologically [understood], that is, based on the truth of be[-ing], and only so!" (*GA* 2, 51, note b). In §83, another note was added following his exact quotation of the definition: "Also nicht Existenzphilosophie": "Thus not philosophy of existing" (*GA* 2, 576, note a). (The passages quoted correspond to the Macquarrie-Robinson translation 38/62 and 436/487, respectively.) Heidegger is certainly referring to Jaspers' philosophy here and perhaps indirectly to Sartre's existentialism, from both of which he distanced himself. The point is that Heidegger's analytics of existence—an ontological pursuit of meaning—should not be confused with analysis (or the appearance of its possessive, 'analytic') of a chemical compound or the psyche, as in psycho-analysis. The latter is an ontic [*ontisch*] affair. On the reference to Aristotle, it is well known that Heidegger's guide through philosophy's hell was Aristotle, for whom the *logos* was approached from what he termed an analytics (prior and posterior), from the Greek ἀναλυτικά, the pursuit of discovering and interpreting a *pattern* of meaning among many things and precisely not something learned by taking apart the structure. The idea of distinguishing the elements of what is a complex whole and revealing its complexity is central to an analytics, but it is different from an analysis.

A. Early Publications Influenced by Martin Heidegger

The second, revised and expanded, edition shows more explicitly the influence of Heidegger's thought. Five years after its appearance, Boss would made clear his debt to Heidegger in his *Psychoanalyse und Daseinsanalytik* (1957). Since 1963 we have known this book in translation as *Psychoanalysis and Daseinsanalysis*. In fact, the two texts have little to do with each other.

By the third edition, Boss and Heidegger had completed the bulk of the Zollikon seminars and they had established a collegial and personal relationship.[1] Additional changes to the text represent the ever-deepening influence of Heidegger. In addition to another new preface, a postscript on the difference between "anthropological psychiatry" (Binswanger) and "daseinsanalytic psychiatry" (Boss) was added. In it, Boss refers to the Zollikon seminars from January 1961 (SG3 180, n. 7) but much more of their influence can be found throughout the revisions. The full influence of Heidegger's thought is patent, as is an explicit repudiation of Binswanger's *Daseinsanalyse*. Binswanger himself eventually admitted to have misunderstood Heidegger (SG3 10). During Boss's lifetime an unchanged 4th edition of the book was issued (1984) which has been reprinted as recently as three years ago (2017).

Some historical and biographical context may be helpful at this point. In 1925, Boss was in analysis with Freud himself during a stay in Vienna financed by his father, who did not, however, pay for the sessions with Freud. In 1927, Heidegger published *Sein und Zeit*. The following year Boss earned his medical degree in Zürich and went on to complete a five-year psychiatric residency with Eugen Bleuler at the Burghölzli Clinic there. Three years before finishing the MD, however, began a training psychoanalysis with Hans Behn-Eschenburg, which lasted for three years. From 1929-1932, Boss continued psychoanalytic studies in Germany and London with prominent analysts including Karen Horney, Hanns Sachs, Wilhelm Reich, Siegfried Bernfeld, Otto Fenichel, and

---

1 There is a photograph of Boss sitting next to Heidegger in Meßkirch on the eve of Heidegger's 70th birthday, two months before their collaboration began with a lecture by Heidegger at the Burghölzli in 1959. Boss's edition of the Zollikon seminars contains several photographs of the two men over the course of their friendship and collaborative work.

A. Early Publications Influenced by Martin Heidegger

Ernest Jones. He was also in professional contact with great neurologist Kurt Goldstein.

In 1938, after an Institute for Psychotherapy was established in Zürich, of which Boss was a founding member, he began a decade-long collegial relationship with Carl Gustav Jung, whom he had met at the Burghölzli.[1] By the time of the book on love was completed, Boss had grown as disenchanted with Jung's revision of Freudian theory (a "psychology of complexes") as with Freud's basic position.

Boss reports that he at last read *Sein und Zeit* in earnest while on military service in the early 1940s. He finally met Heidegger in 1946, after the war had ended and Heidegger was in temporary academic exile. Their meeting at Heidegger's cabin in Todtnauberg, about 70 miles from Zürich, and an ensuing correspondence led to Heidegger's only extended intellectual collaboration with anyone and to what Boss published in 1971 as his *Grudriß der Medizin und der Psychology*, all of which had been carefully edited by Heidegger, who evidently also wrote some sections of the book.

Boss's book on the perversions was his *Habilitationsschrift*, a study completed for the University of Zürich faculty to qualify as a lecturer at the university.[2] It was published in 1947 and bridged his career as a fully trained, card-carrying Freudian psychoanalyst and his reformulation of the ideas of his existential analysis. Much had changed with respect to his understanding of psychoanalysis could be. Boss had already published on psychosomatics, social psychiatry, and marriage, and had eighteen contributions to learned journals to his credit, including one in French. He had written on topics such as the sleep cure in the treatment of schizophrenia, the Rorschach test, electroshock, psychotherapy, and

---

1   These details of Boss's biography are taken from the preface to the English translation of the book (1949) and from Boss's self-portrait written (1973). See my translation, "Médard Boß: A Memoir (1973)," in *Existential Analysis* **30**(1), 2019, pp. 169-198. The details are somewhat at variance with each other in certain places in the preface and the autobiographical sketch.

2   Twenty years earlier, in 1928, as part of earning the title "Dr. med.," Boss wrote a thesis supervised by Hans W. Maier *On the Question of the Evolutionary Biological Significance of Alcohol*. As Alice Holzhey-Kunz pointed out (Personal Communication, June 2019), that was at the time not at all common among individuals who had trained as physicians. He was also reading heavily in Eastern philosophy at the time.

A. Early Publications Influenced by Martin Heidegger

bed wetting (*enuresis nocturna*), as well several articles on topics related to public health policy and his experience as an army doctor during World War II.

The English translation, published two years later, is designated the "second (English language) edition" of the book (MC iv). It is, in fact, a translation of the extensively "expanded and revised" second German edition, which would not be published for three more years. The preface to the second German edition includes a revision of the opening paragraphs of the American version. It is quite brief and Heidegger is only mentioned in passing (SG^2 8). The preface to the American version, however, contains a detailed review of Heidegger's ideas (MC ix-xiii).

This brief biographical and bibliographic excursus makes clear that as originally conceived Boss's *Habilitationsschrift* was already a thing of the past as soon as it was in print in 1947. Boss's thinking was changing dramatically during the year he completed it.[1] The work of a seasoned doctor, psychiatrist and scholar with a pedigree unmatched by any other psychiatrist of his generation, the dissertation was, however, based on Binswanger's mistaken understanding of Heidegger's analytics of existence.

The volume in its successive editions reflects the great distance between the two versions of what came to be known as *Daseinsanalyse*. Most readers assumed they were the same, however, when *Existence. A New Dimension in Psychiatry and Psychology*, edited by Rollo May, Henri Ellenberger and Ernest Angel, was published in 1958. This book, we recall, put existential psychotherapy on the map. It was heavily represented with chapters by Binswanger, but there is nothing in it by Boss. *Existence* and Boss's *Psychoanalyse und Daseinsanalytik* were being prepared for publication at the same time and it could have merely been a matter of timing and snail mail contact between Boss and May. The only English translation of a paper by Boss on the analytics of existence published by 1957 was his "'Daseinsanalysis' and Psychotherapy."[2]

---

[1] Appendix IV compares the first two editions, noting where and the extent to which Heidegger's direct influence, not mediated by Binswanger's early misinterpretation of the analytics of existence, is evident.

[2] In Jules Masserman and J. L. Moreno (eds.), *Progress in Psychotherapy*. Volume II. *Anxiety and Therapy* (New York: Grune and Stratton, 1957), pp. 156-161.

A. Early Publications Influenced by Martin Heidegger

What readers of the "English language" of Boss's book on the paraphilias (if they can find a copy of it now) is all that readers limited to English translations of Boss's work have of his first existential analytical (*daseinsanalytisch*) work.[1] We must take a critical look at the later German editions as well both the introduction by Oskar Diethelm and Boss's preface to the 1949 translation in order to see how his thinking and practice changed. On the other hand, if we examine only the English translation, we may appreciate why his reception among English-speaking psychiatrists was as minimal as it was.

The context and background of Boss's book on the paraphilias may not be evident to younger readers. Therefore, before looking at the two prefaces and the third edition's postscript, a word is in order about Boss and gender, a theme central to his book on love and paraphilias.

So much has changed even since the late 1960s, when this book on other sexualities was given its final form. For example, homosexuality was voted out as a psychological disorder by the American Psychiatric Association in 1973 and we have long since stopped speaking in terms of perversions. Even the category "sexual disorders" was abandoned for the *DSM-5* (2013).

While the subtitle is significant for containing the word *daseinsanalytisch*, it is just as surprising for the appearance of the word *Liebe* (love) in it. Boss writes about sex and love—not about gender. When he uses the word *Geschlecht* he has in mind only biological sex and sexual behavior, not gender. When he uses the word 'love' he has in mind both physical and emotional intimacy, sometimes in combination and often even with an implicit spiritual element. During Boss's formative years the notion of gender in its contemporary sense was nonexistent. The only meaning of gender was in grammar where it referred to masculine, feminine, and neuter nouns. The term as used in its current sense was introduced into academic discussions by,

---

Reprinted in Hendrik Ruitenbeek (ed.) *Psychoanalysis and Existential Philosophy* (New York: Dutton, 1962), pp. 81-89. Full bibliographic information on this an all works by Boss will be found in my International Bibliography of the Writings of Medard Boss (1929-2003) found at the end of this volume.

1 Note that *daseinsanalytisch* translates as both existential-analytic when referring to the psychotherapy modality *Daseinsanalyse* and existential-analytical when referring to Heidegger's *Daseinsanalytik*. This is a peculiarity of German that has caused a number of mix-ups. See the Glossary.

A. Early Publications Influenced by Martin Heidegger

among others, the American anthropologist Margaret Mead, the British sociologist Alex Comfort, and the American psychiatrist Harry Stack Sullivan. It eventually reached English-speaking psychiatrists, who gradually incorporated it into their understanding of sexual psychopathology and just at a time when the theme was becoming politically charged. That is still its status, even though some (the author included) believe we are now entering a post-gender era in which a fundamental biological understanding of sex is regaining hegemony.[1]

Boss's account of the perversions is more than a study of parasexualities (my neologism) and reflects the literal meaning of the term that would soon replace it: paraphilias (other forms of *love*). On the other hand, it would likely not pass muster today because he understood the parasexualities in terms of deficiency, but not regression, which was the view of the sexologists whose works he studied, especially Wilhelm von Krafft-Ebing's *Psychopathia Sexualis* (1886). For these men, homosexuality and the other perversions were evidence of degeneration—literally, an evolutionary step back in certain individuals from the level humanity had attained, namely, default heterosexuality. Boss's position was that heterosexuality is the most fulfilling expression of being human in which emotional intimacy and physical contact between two human beings, one male and one female, occurs and attains its fullest realization.[2] Boss did not believe that individuals

---

[1] The politicization of psychiatry as the handmaiden of legislators and the judicial system has moved some of us, following Thomas Szasz and others, to question whether any real gains in understanding the paraphilias and their treatment have resulted from having introduced the now significant distinction between biological sex and psychosocial gender. We can all agree, however, that the distinction has become a dominant concern for parents, educators, counselors and psychotherapists, and physicians, including psychiatrists. Something similar can be said about the connection between politics and psychiatry. For this, everything published by Thomas Szasz is relevant. See also David Healy, *The Creation of Psychopharmacology* (Cambridge: Harvard University Press, ²2004, revised edition).

[2] Apart from a handful of rare genetic anomalies, there are only two sexes, male and female, representatives of which are, respectively, a man(-person) and a woman(-person). The English words 'male' and 'female' look as though they are related etymologically, so that that the one word with a prefix (fe-male) might be based on the other (male). They are not so related. On the other hand, 'man' and 'woman' are, with the prefix 'wo-' designating that the 'wo-man' is a *wife* of the 'man'. The word 'man' is both generic for "human being" ('Man', in German *Mensch*,

A. Early Publications Influenced by Martin Heidegger

displaying other sexualities were subhuman, but only less fully expressive of their potentiality for intimate experience with others. Their capacity for expression was constricted, but they were not depraved as the nineteenth-century sexologists had suggested. Boss always saw sex and love as united if sexuality was genuinely human. This view, as every reader knows, is highly contested in our time.

On the other hand, for Boss, the emotional dimension of heterosexual intimacy could be experienced without physical contact and the same held for his eight case examples of parasexualities. Psychiatric psychopathology in these cases did not entail moral disapproval, implicit in the forensic psychiatry that had been outlined by the sexologists. The pervert was not a "bad" person like a felon. Prior to (*jenseits*) good and evil, that is, understood from the perspective of the analytics of existence, psychopathological behavior has to do only with the *limited realization* of possibilities inherent to existence. Of course, every instance of existence is limited by the givens of natural and historical context and situation. Boss is concerned with potentialities and unrealized possibilities. This is especially important for considerations of his existential analysis as therapy.

Boss's famous counter to Freud's "Why?"—a question about etiology and answered by hypotheses of causation—was "Why not?" That meant setting conditions in which the freedom of the individual might be least encumbered. Any instance of psychopathology, as in the perversions, was an instance of freedom limited.

The upshot of this for a psychiatry of other sexualities *à la* Boss is that we must begin with a view of human *being*—existence—that is more basic than the one promulgated by the natural (and social) sciences. For Boss, to understand norm (heterosexuality) and deprivation (the paraphilic or perverse), it is necessary to take a view of the other there facing me, meeting me as and within a range of possibility,

---

when *man* is the indefinite "one" or "they") and an indication of an instance of *homo sapiens sapiens* with an XY set of sex chromosomes. The sex chromosomes of a 'wo-man' are XX. Those of a 'man' are XY, which indicates the absence of some genetic material. (The 'Y' is an 'X' with its lower right piece missing). The irony in all this for "gender studies" is that, embryologically, all human beings are initially sexually undifferentiated. Here is existence *in utero*.

A. Early Publications Influenced by Martin Heidegger

and not, for example, as a personality of one type or another with a given set of traits.[1]

All this is to remind the reader that Boss's book is about love and sex understood normatively as occurring together or in some cases when there is love without sex. It is not about gender, which allows for genital and other apparent expressions of sexuality (foreplay, anal intercourse) without real intimacy and as more or less mechanical responses not unlike elimination, coughing or sneezing.

Before turning to the "second (English language) edition," readers should be familiar with the German preface to the other second German edition. It is translated here for the first time:

"Preface" to the 2nd German Edition (1952)[2]

[7] The great interest which this book met in the world of scientific psychology and psychopathology, and the importance attached to it by its critics, compelled me to think through all those passages in the preparation of its second edition the formulation of which I was not unequivocally sure had been successful. I finally found myself forced to make two expansions of the original text. For one thing, it seemed to me that this helped in understanding my intentions to present the current path of development of the theories on sexual perversions in more detail. That is, what I hoped to make even clearer is how this path leads from classical psychoanalytic psychophysics to its transformation into a psychoanalytic ego psychology, on the one hand, and to the views of the so-called anthropological investigators, on the other hand, to the existential-analytical viewpoint. Now, from the outset, the serious misunderstanding must have become impossible that the existential-analytical approach would mean a relapse into a mere "consciousness psychology" and would be "hostile" to the psychoanalytic conception based on unconscious material. In actuality, the

---

1 Once disburdened of Freud's metapsychology, modern psychiatry developed into a system in which psychopathology is diagnosed on the basis of the notion of personality. This is the real legacy of humanistic psychology, beginning with Gordon Allport and his trait psychology.
2 See Appendix I for the German text. Page numbers corresponding to it are given in brackets.

A. Early Publications Influenced by Martin Heidegger

existential-analytical approach considers "the preconscious" and "the unconscious" no less than anything already known by the patient. Precisely for this reason, however, it is able to include all earlier insights and form a basis for understanding that supports them as partial aspects.

So, too, the fact that more and more the usual psychoanalytic terminology was avoided should no longer encourage this misunderstanding. For the more open, more cautious existential-analytical idiom was preferred only because psychoanalytic theory with its abstract concepts of an "id," an "ego," a "superego," etc., all too easily seduces us into a dangerous objectification, reification, and artificial dismemberment of man. Of course, classical psychoanalytic *praxis* and technique are not at all [8] affected by these objections. To me it has always proved itself to be for my patients, whose pathologically determined upsetting experience of the world and of themselves is for the most part consistently unknown to them, the unsurpassable method to make their determining basic feelings more palpable to them and thereby make them therapeutically more susceptible. In the first part of the book I also added the section "Psychological Remarks on the Norm of Love." I tried to relate the phenomena of loving even more originally to the structures of the essence of human existence as they have been sketched out for us by Martin Heidegger. The deeper the insights into the essence of human love are able to penetrate, the wider the horizon of understanding of the phenomena of sexual perversions opens up.

The second part of the book, in which the concrete individual fate of sexually perverse people are described, I was able to leave for the most part unchanged. All the sexually perverted patients into whose lives psychoanalytic praxis has allowed me to gain insight since the publication of the first edition have brought me only further complete confirmation of these case presentations.

Zürich, Spring 1951
M. Boss

"Preface" to the "Second (English language) Edition" (1949)

The first "second edition" was published in English two years before the second, German "second edition." Since this book is the first Boss

A. Early Publications Influenced by Martin Heidegger

had translated into English, what is said about key terms in its preface is especially important for what readers would come to expect when his next books to be translated, on dreams (1958; German, 1953) and on psychoanalysis and Heidegger's analytics of existence (1963; German, 1957), were published.

The material unique to the translation (MC x-xii) may have been based on a manuscript Boss wrote in German that was then translated in conformity with the translator's decisions about key terms. There is no German text to consult, since Boss's *Nachlaß* is not yet available and the publisher is no longer in business. It is also possible that Boss wrote it in English and the translator either published it as given to him or subsequently touched it up. It is certain that he considered the translation of key terms and passed them along to the translator, but the resulting text was not helpful: "The term *daseinsanalysis* appearing throughout this work results from a problem in semantics. The German *Daseinsanalyse* translates readily as *existential analysis*; however, the English term *existential* has assumed, particularly following World War II, connotations that may be misleading here. My own use of the term relates to my own experience with it." Some details of his early experience, already recounted above, follow.

There is evidence that Boss did not write the preface and did not see it before the book was published. The publication date of *Sein und Zeit* is given incorrectly as 1929. *Seiende*, seemingly glossing "human individuals" is misspelled.

Here are the relevant passages:

> In 1929 [sic] Martin Heidegger published his fundamental ontology in his basic work "Sein und Zeit," and he himself called it [a] "Daseinsanalytik" (existential analysis)....
>
> Martin Heidegger's existential analysis has become the basis of my own thinking in psychopathology. For the first time since the ancient age of the Greeks Heidegger as a philosopher has differentiated clearly between the [?] non-objectifying "being" (Sein), which cannot be grasped sensually, and the [?] concrete "beings," the things, animals and human individuals (Seindes) [sic] in which the former appears in thousand-fold forms and shapes in which it manifests itself.

A. Early Publications Influenced by Martin Heidegger

Great credit is due to Ludwig Binswanger who has introduced into psychiatry this daseinsanalytic mode of thinking of Heidegger, and who has pointed out its revolutionizing significance for psychopathology. In [?] one point, however, I do not agree with Binswanger. In his important book on "Grundformern und Erkenntnis menschlichen Daseins" he not only feels that he has to augment and change Heidegger's conception [?] by adding most careful investigations on the [?] human love but there he tries to extract from Heidegger's fundamental ontology an anthropology, an isolated theory of man. Martin Heidegger himself believes this to be impossible.

The most important mishap here is translating Heidegger's *Daseinsanaltik* with "existential analysis" which sets a precedent for confusing Heidegger's analytics of existence with existential analysis as a form of psychotherapy. As Boss knew, Binswanger's "daseinsanalytic mode of thinking" (based on the his *Daseinsanalyse*) was not Heidegger's daseinsanalytical procedure (based on the *Daseinsanalytik* project in *Being and Time*), but this is obscured.

Boss then takes up Sartre's misappropriation of Heidegger's *Daseinanaltik* and mentions the latter's confirmation "personally in a recent discussion" of Sartre's error. He concludes: "Therefore my daseinsanalytic thinking has nothing whatsoever to do with Sartre's existentialism," characterized earlier as "famous and infamous." He reaffirms: "Heidegger himself has stated to me personally that my thinking has understood correctly the essence and core of his conceptions." In this passage, Boss is evidently using an adjectival form of *Daseinsanalyse*, although he has alerted the reader to Sartre's error by referring to the *Daseinsanalytik*.

Now we come to what is most problematic, and perhaps, in part, the most egregious influence on subsequent translators of Boss's later publications: "Unfortunately, 'Da-sein' in the sense in which Heidegger uses it cannot be translated into the English language without employing lengthy and cumbersome circumscriptions."[1] Here and from here

---

1 Martin Heidegger, *Existence and Being* (Chicago: Henry Regnery, 1949), edited by Werner Brock, with translations by R.F.C. Hull, Alan Crick and Douglas Scott. It was Brock who correctly translated *Daseinsanalytik* as "analytics of Dasein."

A. Early Publications Influenced by Martin Heidegger

on out, it would have made sense to render *Dasein* with 'existence' and, sensibly, formulations such as analysis of existence (*Daseinsanalyse*) and analytics of existence (*Daseinsanalytik*) would have followed.

The first translations of Heidegger in English, *Existence and Being*, appeared the same year as the translation of Boss's book. It would be

---

Dasein remained untranslated but was glossed with "human life." Brock also frequently used the phrase "human Dasein," which is redundant. *Da-sein* (hyphenated) is rendered with "being there" or "There being," reflecting the decision of R.F.C. Hull and Alan Crick in their translation of *Vom Wesen der Wahrheit* [*On the Essence of Truth*], which had been published only in 1943. In a note, the translators and editor freely exchange *Da-sein* for *Dasein*, which was surely an error. Readers will recall the note on the word *Dasein* by John Macquarrie and Edward Robinson in their translation of *Sein und Zeit*: "The word 'Dasein' plays so important a role in this work and is already so familiar to the English-speaking reader who has read about Heidegger, that it seems simpler to leave it untranslated except in the relatively rare passages in which Heidegger himself breaks it up with a hyphen ('Da-sein') to show its etymological construction: literally 'Being-there.'" *Being and Time* (New York: Harper and Row, 1962), p. 27, n. 1. (Cf. p. 172, where the translators render the hyphenated form with 'Being-there' and set the stage for Chapter 5, especially on Being-there (not Dasein, as usual) as "state-of-mind [*Befindlichkeit*]," "understanding [*Verstehen*]," and "discourse [*Rede*]," and "the everyday be[-]ing of the there." This bears reflection given that the Joan Stambaugh translation includes the following observation: "It was Heidegger's express wish that in future translations the word *Da-sein* should be hyphenated throughout *Being and Time*, a practice he himself instigated, for example, in chapter 5 of Division One." *Being and Time* (Albany: SUNY Press, 1996), p. xiv. In his revision (2010) of the Stambaugh translation, Dennis Schmidt undoes this. In fact, apart from in his notes to the *Complete Edition* edition (1977), Heidegger hyphenates the word fairly infrequently outside of the chapter mentioned, where he is focusing on the existentive [*existenzial*] constitution of the there [*da*] as such. It makes sense there to visualize that element of the term. Reflecting on the Macquarrie/Robinson note, one wonders about the "familiarity" of the reader with leaving 'Dasein' untranslated. Apart from *Existence and Being* only four books of translations had been published before *Being and Time* appeared in 1962, and the first two were bilingual, which provided the reader with some guidance: *What Is Philosophy?* (1958) (translated by William Kluback and Jeanne T. Wilde), *The Question of Being* (1958) (translated by William Kluback and Jeanne T. Wilde), *An Introduction to Metaphysics* (1959) (translated by Ralph Mannheim, and *Essays in Metaphysics: Identity and Difference* (1960) (translated by Kurt Leidecker). In any case, Mannheim had translated *Dasein* with 'being-there'; Kluback and Wilde had used both 'reality' and 'existence' for *Dasein* in *The Question of Being* and 'actuality' for *Dasein* in *What Is Philosophy?* Leidecker translated the word with 'existence'.

A. Early Publications Influenced by Martin Heidegger

another thirteen years before *Being and Time* was published. *Existence and Being* was the author's first exposure to Heidegger, as it was for most English-speaking readers. Looking back to the long summary of *Sein und Zeit* by Werner Brock, I am sure that, like Boss, Heidegger in English was mostly incomprehensible to us. On *Dasein*, the editor and translators wrote: "It is proposed to leave this key-term as a *terminus technicus heideggerianus*," chiefly because of the tendency of readers to think of *Dasein* in its common everyday meaning as existence (as in "the existence of God") (p. 397, n. 15). But, untutored in German, English readers would not have been sensitive to this. In any case, the word has been left untranslated for the most part ever since, including in the term *Daseinsanalyse*.

While Boss's view of Freud would change dramatically over the next few years, especially arguing against the coherence of the notion of transference, in 1947, however, he still adhered to the basic *therapeutic* principles of classic psychoanalysis. "I need not regard myself as a dissenter from Freud, certainly not with respect to the practice of [?] my treatment of neuroses and of perversions."

Boss's reference to the "new way of anthropologic thinking, which Heidegger has taught us" is puzzling since only a few sentences earlier he had made it plain that an anthropology could not be "extracted" from Heidegger's ontology.

We move now to the preface to the third edition of Boss's book on love. By now, many sessions of the Zollikon seminars were under his belt. His closeness to Heidegger's ideas is central to the text. It is presented here in translation for the first time. I have **bolded** the most important passages and allow them to speak for themselves.

"Preface" to the 3rd German Edition (1966)

[9] Twenty years have passed since the days when this book was first printed. In the course of such a long time, the author has seen dozens of new patients suffering from sexual perversions. Some of them he has treated himself. Most of them were patients whose therapy was carried out by his pupils, all under his constant supervision.

Not a single one of these twenty years of experience has contradicted in any fundamental way the meaning and content of sexual

A. Early Publications Influenced by Martin Heidegger

perversions described in the first edition of the book. This may well be a convincing proof of the validity of the insights gained at that time.

On the other hand, it would testify to an unpardonable intellectual inertia on the author's part if in the meantime he had not been able to obtain an even more accurate intellectual formulation and clearer foundation of the facts he saw two decades earlier. **Meaning and Content of Sexual Perversions came about as the very first fruit of the contact in my medical-psychiatric experience with the new understanding of man that we owe to Martin Heidegger's philosophical analytics of existence. The conflict of psychiatry with the analytics of existence that had lasted for three decades was characterized by some fundamental and extremely confusing misunderstandings on the part of doctors, especially at the beginning.**

The blame for these misunderstandings was, above all, the aftereffect of Husserl's "phenomenology" on medical representatives of the newly emerging "psychiatric analytics of existence." Husserl's "phenomenology," however, is one of ego consciousness and thus remains attached to the idea of man as a subjectivity. On the other hand, **the all-defining conception of human being as "existence," as Heidegger crystallized it in his analytics of existence, is in sharpest contrast to it all about breaking up this subjectivist conception, better yet, not letting it first arise.**

Continual misunderstanding of the ontological determinations of human being in Heidegger's analytics of existence as ontic assertions about human behavior was to blame for the confusing misunderstandings of the early "existential-analytic" psychiatrists. From such confusion stemmed the impossibility of a clarified understanding of the relationship between essential, ontological statements about human being and ontic, psychiatrically determinable human phenomena.

Fortunately, the necessary clarification of this psychiatric confusion has taken place in recent years from both of the solely relevant sides. To begin with, in 1958 Ludwig Binswanger, who has the lasting merit of being the first to have called to the attention of psychiatrists the epoch-making of Martin Heidegger's work, ventured the extremely courageous public admission that he had misunderstood Heidegger's

A. Early Publications Influenced by Martin Heidegger

thinking. As a result, Binswanger has since then also consistently made the terms "existential analysis" and "existential-analytic", taken from Heidegger's work *Sein und Zeit* at that time, the designation for his own work and from then on only referred to Husserl's "phenomenology". With such rare restrained scientific and human courage Binswanger has as far as possible called a halt to the further proliferation of a confusion that was bound to have come about, especially among students, since, initially, identical designations were used for two completely different views of the fundamental essence of man.

On the other hand, aspiring psychiatrists in Zürich have been receiving regular seminars for about five years which Heidegger himself holds twice or three times a semester in in collaboration with the author of this work in Zollikon [11]. On these occasions, Heidegger never tires of confirming to psychiatrists that what Ludwig Binswanger introduced into psychiatry has nothing to do with his understanding of the analytics of existence. Rather, there could be no greater error than that committed by Binswanger in his characterization of the analytics of existence as an extremely consistent continuation of the teachings of Kant and Husserl.

In this way, then, it has been made clear with all desirable clarity by the two most competent authorities just what kind of psychiatric work has anything to do with Heidegger's analytics of existence and his singular existential analysis and that which cannot be associated with his view, which is also why the designation 'existential-analytic' does not at all appertain to the matter since it was devised by its creator for a completely different thinking and way of seeing.

Because this is beyond any doubt, it is to be expected that soon the commendable procedure of L. Binswanger will be followed by his students only with hesitation. In the near future they will no longer call their scientific work "existential-analytic" method of working, but will try to find another name instead.

Given such a frank concession of the different nature of their method of investigation from that of Heidegger's analytics of existence a clean, also well-established terminological differentiation from the existential-analytical approach to psychopathological phenomena cannot be difficult for them and, in fact, on this basis psychiatric existential analysis is not prejudiced in the slightest with regard to any

A. Early Publications Influenced by Martin Heidegger

possible qualitative difference of the appropriateness of one or the another view in terms of its fruitfulness for what psychiatry is about.

Naturally, preparations for the third edition of *Meaning and Content of Sexual Perversions* were not permitted to ignore the significant events that took place in the field of psychiatry in the course of the past decade, as **Heidegger was engaged in a personal, ongoing discussion with the discipline of psychiatry in order to accomplish with unprecedented precision a decisive differentiation in it between two fundamental issues. Now it is clearer than ever before that the philosophical-ontological analysis of existence [Daseinsanalyse] and its being carried out in the form of the singular ontological analysis of existence, as worked out in *Being and Time*, is to be distinguished from an ontic existential-analytic psychopathology and its implementation by means of descriptions and interpretations of concrete, psychologically ascertainable human ways of behaving which as such are on the horizon of that very philosophical ontological analytics of existence and existential analysis.**

All of these fundamental clarifications regarding the relation between philosophy and psychiatry made a substantial revision of the first chapters of the present book unavoidable, since they aim at a determination of the essence of the normative human capacity for loving. Such a fundamental reflection was imperative from the start, so that the following sections dealing with psychopathological phenomena of love would not remain up in the air, but rather be built on solid ground. Properly speaking, all unhealthy behavior is only a deficient appearance of normative possibilities of relating and to be understood as the want of health. As a phenomenon of privation, as a deficient state of health, everything that is pathological always and necessarily remains related to the normative, healthy human being as its basis. The normative capacity for loving is in turn always only one of the possible means of fulfillment of human being as a whole. Therefore, for a correct understanding of normative as well as all pathological intimate behavior [13], an insight into the essential traits, into the specific mode of being, the basic nature of being human in general is the indispensable prerequisite. In other words, in all psychological-psychiatric research it is also always necessary to first bring clarity

A. Early Publications Influenced by Martin Heidegger

with regard to an adequately ontological determination. All factually ascertainable human behavior is always and constantly overseen in advance by the ontological determination of the essential traits of human being as what is most proper to it. Therefore, there must never be easy talk of wanting to separate ontological thinking from ontic-psychiatric observing and interpreting, and of leaving that entirely to the philosopher.

Of course, the proper elaboration and making transparent the ontological determinations of human being is and remains the task of essential thinkers, the philosophers, and can never be the business of medical psychopathologists or scientific psychologists. Therefore, **all psychologists and psychiatrists, including all sex pathologists, depend on this fundamental preparatory work of the thinker.** It bears witness to a profoundly dangerous denial of the psychology and psychiatry authors' own potential for superficiality, when a psychiatric point of view is accused again and again of moving strictly within the horizon of essential insights that have to thank for them the thinking of a philosopher.

Relatively few changes due to the revision of the introductory chapter were necessary, however, in the area of presentation of eight concrete case histories of sexually perverse people that follows the general part of the book. After all, the new formulations are incisive enough so that it is to be hoped that they will also allow the meaning and content of the sexual perversions as taken from the patients themselves and presented in their essential meaning in the first edition to stand out even more clearly and vividly now.

August, 1966
Medard Boss

In the preface, Boss traces problems of understanding among psychiatrists following Binswanger and Binswanger's own misunderstanding of Heidegger to their having failed, with Husserl (and Freud, we might add), to transcend the reification of consciousness as a subject or ego, something that Heidegger had accomplished. He also praises Binswanger for having admitted the error of his ways.

A. Early Publications Influenced by Martin Heidegger

The Zollikon seminars, in which the difference between the two sorts of *Daseinsanalyse* were made explicit, Boss is optimistic that a "well-established terminological differentiation" had been made between the two approaches. That, sad to say, seems not to have happened. Finally, Boss highlights the philosophical basis of his approach. Would that other psychotherapists were able to see each approach has a philosophical foundation. Freud's own distaste for philosophy comes to mind here. We cannot avoid thinking that psychoanalysis could only have benefitted from Freud's having made explicit its metaphysics.

The third edition concludes with an important postscript. My translation of it follows next. Once again, I have **bolded** the passages relevant to our discussion. It is remarkable that Boss's critic, Viktor von Gebsattel, who is discussed was for a period of time Heidegger's psychiatrist. Heidegger had this to say about his treatment: "And what did [von Gebsattel] do? He just started walking randomly with me through the snow-covered winter forest. He did not do anything else. But as a human being he helped me, so that three weeks later I was again healthy and returned home."[1]

"Postscript" to the 3rd German Edition (1966)

[174] Not long after the publication of the second edition of the preceding treatise the most outspoken representative of the so-called "anthropological theory of perversions," [Viktor] von Gebsattel,

---

1   See my "Medard Boss's Daseinsanalysis of Martin Heidegger. Reflections and a Conjecture on an Unexplored Aspect of the Zollikon Seminars," in *Existential Analysis* **26**(2), 2015, p. 271. Heidegger expressed his thanks to von Gebsattel in 1958 by publishing a lecture he had given the previous year, "Principles of Thinking," in the *Jahrbuch für Psychologie und Psychotherapie* (Freiburg) 6, 1958, pp. 33-41. I am reminded of R.D. Laing's observation that in therapy, the *treatment* (the cure or course of therapy) is nothing more or less than the way the therapist *treats* the person, that is, "the way he acts towards" the person. In his last paper, von Gebsattel wrote about the highest (third) stage of patient-doctor interaction as occurring at the level of "spiritual-pastoral" and "spiritual-medical" acts. "The Meaning of Medical Practice," in *Theoretical Medicine* **14**(1), 1995, p. 70 (translated by Jos V.M. Welie). Von Gebsattel traces his insight into the third phase of therapeutic encounter to Kierkegaard (p. 70). He was among the physicians of his time who had strong ties to Catholicism. Perhaps this was brought "home" to Heidegger in their interactions.

A. Early Publications Influenced by Martin Heidegger

honored our criticism of his view with a reply to it in a chapter that appeared in his *Prolegomena to a Medical Anthropology* published in 1954.[1] There, with keen insight, he recognized that "the dispute over the correctness of the existential-analytical or anthropological theory is more accurately one about the *symbolic value* of the perverse acts which are fully grasped or not fully grasped in their special structure" (p. 218).

[175] But with nothing else than this "argument" that wants to let a *symbolic value* allegedly contained in perverse acts decide about the correctness or incorrectness of his view, von Gebsattel has only been able to prove more conclusively how little he has considered in his theory the phenomena experienced by patients themselves and attended to the contents of meaning and referential contexts that are inherently associated with and actually form them. For what is the so-called *symbolic value* of a matter anything other than the cognitive-emotional content an observer attributes as an addition and from his "unconscious psyche" appends "psychologically" to the so-called pure factuality of a phenomenon? The entirely unbridgeable gap between all subjectivist anthropological theories and the special approach of an existential-analytical phenomenological study of humanity is palpable in such a "symbolic" approach. There is nothing more suitable to revealing the existential-analytical phenomenological method of investigation, which pervaded throughout and determined in every detail by it made the present work possible in the first place, and to delineating its essence and making manifest what it is and what it wants to be than a clarification of precisely the gap that separates it from all "anthropological" theories. Regarding that, **let us first mention the characterization of so-called symbolic values and contents that we owe to M. Heidegger.**

---

1 "Daseinsanalytische und anthropologische Auslegung der sexuellen Perversionen [Existential-Analytical and Anthropological Interpretation of Sexual Perversions]," in *Prolegomena einer medizinischen Anthropologie* (Berlin: Springer, 1955), pp. 212-220. The essay is the eighth of twenty papers published by von Gebsattel. In this essay, he speaks of the beginning of the patient-doctor partnership as the physician's response to a "call," of the practice of medicine as a calling. The essays range from fetishism and depersonalization to the anthropology of *Angst*.

A. Early Publications Influenced by Martin Heidegger

In his essay "Building Dwelling Thinking," in order to make clear the richness of contents of meaning inherent in the thing itself Heidegger describes a bridge. Concerning it, he recalls: "The bridge swings over the stream 'with ease and power.' It does not merely connect shores that are already there. The shores emerge as shores only as the bridge crosses the stream. By design, the bridge causes them to lie across from each other. One side [176] is set off against the other by the bridge. Nor do the shores stretch along the stream as indifferent strips of bordering dry land. With shores the bridge brings to the stream one and the other expanse of landscape lying behind them. It brings stream and shore and land into each other's neighborhood. The bridge *gathers* the earth as landscape around the stream. Thus it leads it through the meadows. Resting upright in the stream bed, the bridge piers bear the swing of the arches that let the stream's waters run their course.... [/] The bridge lets the stream run its course and at the same time grants to mortals their way, so that they might come and go from place to place. Bridges convey in many ways. The city bridge leads from the precincts of the castle to the cathedral square; the river bridge near the country town brings horse-drawn wagons to the surrounding villages. The nondescript brook crossing of the old stone bridge gives the harvest wagon passage from the fields into the village and carries the lumber cart from the field path to the road. The highway bridge is tied into a network of roads for calculated and fastest possible long-distance travel. Always and ever differently, the bridge conveys the hesitant and hasty ways of men to and fro, so that they may get to other shores and, in the end, as mortals, to the other side. Now through a high arc, now through a low, the bridge vaults glen and stream, whether mortals keep in mind this vaulting of the bridge's course or forget that they themselves, always already on their way to the last bridge, are actually striving to surmount their banality and misery in order to bring themselves before the healing of the godly. The bridge *gathers* as the vaulting passage of the godly. Whether their presence be expressly thought of and visibly *given thanks for*, as in the figure of the saint of the bridges, whether it be disguised or entirely displaced."

Given such a grasp of the bridge in its distinct and complete context of meaning and reference, it is easy for [177] Heidegger to correct the

A. Early Publications Influenced by Martin Heidegger

"symbolic" error of today's psychologies. He continues in the same passage: "To be sure, people think of the bridge as primarily and really *just* a bridge. Later and on occasion it might express much more besides. As such an expression, it would then become a symbol, for example, of all the things mentioned before. But the bridge, if it is a real bridge, is never first of all merely a bridge and then afterwards a symbol, in the sense that it expresses something that, strictly speaking, does not belong to it. If we take the bridge strictly as such, it never appears as an expression. The bridge is a thing and *only this*.... [/] Of course, our thinking has long been accustomed to formulate the nature of the thing *too poorly*. In the course of Western thought, the consequence has been that the thing is represented as an unknown X to which perceptible properties are attached. From this point of view, everything *that already belongs to the gathering essence of this thing* does, of course, appear as an additional something subsequently read into it."[1]

In principle, just as with the "psychological symbolizations" of a bridge, the search for the "symbol value," which in the opinion of anthropological psychopathologists secretly accrues to the sexual behavior of sexually perverse people, arises from too poor an assessment of the very essence of this behavior itself. If we only let this speak to us through the mouth of the patient, like all sexual behavior in general it tells us of its own fundamental essence, never of nihilism and destruction, but always of expansion, unification, augmentation, of victory over ordinary configurations.

In the second place, we must content ourselves with referring to [178] those statements by G. Condrau in 1965 in which that author had already anticipated and carried out our critique of the criticism of v. Gebsattel.[2]

Condrau writes, we deem with full justification: "In a way, the existential analysis of Boss is closer than Kunz to the 'anthropological'

---

1 Boss's note: M. Heidegger, ["Bauen Wohnen Denken," in] *Vorträge und Aufsätze*, 1954, 153 ff. For a critique of the psychological concept of the symbol, see also M. Boss, *The Dream and Its Interpretation*, 1953, 96 ff.
2 Boss's note: G. Condrau, *Die Daseinsanalyse von Medard Boß und ihre Bedeutung für die Psychiatrie* [*The Existential Analysis of Medard Boss and Its Significance for Psychiatry*], 1965, 80 ff.

A. Early Publications Influenced by Martin Heidegger

psychiatrist V. E. v. Gebsattel. However, he also has much to find fault with in the approach of existential analysis. His critique is directed in particular against the existential-analytical understanding of the essence and sense of the sexual perversions. In this area, it appears to him that "a revision of existential-analytical theory ... [is] required."[1] Von Gebsattel also adds that if Boss[2] sees a clear manifestation of love in its perverse impoverished and mutilating forms, this assessment of sexual intercourse and orgasm thus appears to be naïve and without question represents the weak point of the new existential-analytical theory of perversions.[3]

To Boss's naively formulated qualification von Gebsattel opposes his own "anthropological" interpretation, which seeks to recognize in all sexually perverse acts the "*disposition and tendency toward evil*—or if from an anthropological perspective we want to avoid this moral theological sounding phrase—*the fundamentally nihilistic inclination of human nature.*" Boss is accused of simply overlooking that in man there is also "a libidinal desire to destroy, to destruction as such," and that this is given symbolic expression everywhere in the sexual perversions.[4]

As entirely unquestionable as von Gebsattel wishes it to be, however, scarcely any authority on the matter agrees with this claim of the critic. Admittedly, Boss will let himself be called entirely "naïve" [179] if beneath it all von Gebsattel understands his approach as one that seeks to dwell on the content of meaning and referential contexts of a given phenomenon encountered by a person so as to let these be there to appear and be perceived intact and directly on their own. Given these efforts of his on behalf of a phenomenological approach to things, Boss knows himself to be guilt free precisely of any demonstrable moments of degrading what is under consideration to something "symbolically" expressed, which is necessarily inherent in von Gebsattel's "anthropological" interpretation. For

---

1 Condrau's note: V. Gebsattel, "Prolegomena einer medizinischen Anthropologie", Berlin, Göttingen, Heidelberg, 1954, p. 220.
2 For the rest of Postscript Boss refers to himself in the third person, suggesting that he is simply paraphrasing what can be found in Condrau's book.
3 Boss's note: *Loc. cit.*, 217.
4 Boss's note: *Loc. cit.*, 219.

A. Early Publications Influenced by Martin Heidegger

while he inquires about an enigmatic "symbolic value" of the sexually perverse act, from the outset he always allows it to be only something derived, derived no matter which way precisely from something behind the phenomenon, thought to be attributable to strivings, "dispositions" and "inclinations" tapped into.[1]

So far, over months and years of psychoanalytic observation of sexually perverted people by Boss and his students, without exception neither the patients themselves nor their analysts ever recognized upfront a primordial "propensity to evil" or a "fundamentally nihilistic trait of human nature" in connection with the pathological behavior associated with their "naïve," immediate self-experience. To the contrary, sexual life even up to orgasm is experienced by these patients invariably and entirely as having the significance of overcoming boundaries, to experience a "beyond oneself," even though in the meantime they lack the inherent redemptive [180] liberation and expansiveness fostered by a normative act of love. In other words, this means that every single perverse sexual act is by no means qualitatively different from normative love, but merely represents its *privative* appearance. However, a privation is fundamentally anything but the negation of being "robbed" of something, of lacking something. Accordingly, even less so with privation is the meaning and content of a phenomenon turned into its opposite. Rather, every privative phenomenon rightly points to the full content of the meaning of the intact manifestation. And so, for example, every shadow is by no means the opposite of what is bright. The shadow only lacks a bit of what is bright. Precisely thanks to this privative feature every shadow also belongs then to the content of the meaning of "brightness."

If v. Gebsattel wants to devalue Boss's very careful concrete observations of patients that the cases presented are not entirely perverse, not to be called drive aberrant psychopaths, this objection is easy to ward off. With the exception of two of the sexually perverted patients cited, from the clinical psychiatric side of things all the others were classified as entirely drive aberrant psychopaths. Therefore should this objection of v. Gebsattel's carry any weight the critic really must present concrete case histories of equally carefully examined sexual

---

[1] Boss's note: Cf. M. Boss, *Introduction to Psychosomatic Medicine*, 1957, 87.

A. Early Publications Influenced by Martin Heidegger

perverts whose self-experience is directly attributable to v. Gebsattel's "interpretation of symbols."

So far, however, instead of concrete, direct evidence in the form of the self-experience of sexually perverse people, we find in v. Gebsattel's criticism only the assertion that it would be necessary to adopt his "anthropological theory of perversions" [181] from the "point of view of an anthropology," which ascribes to the image of man categories other than those developed by Boss.

It is of benefit to consider the validity of this second "argument" against the existential-analytic understanding of the sexual perversions on the basis of **Heidegger's statements on the nature of modern anthropologies in general, which one may read in the essay "The Age of the World View."** [1] He begins by pointing out that in **all of today's anthropologies there is that philosophical interpretation of man which explains and assesses all that is there starting with man and ending with man.** This characterization is elucidated later as follows: **"Anthropology is that interpretation of man which already knows, fundamentally, who man is and therefore can never ask who he is. For it would have to confess itself to be shaken and overcome by this question. How is this to be expected of anthropology when its task is expressly and nothing other than to provide the safeguards that follow from the self-confidence of the** subiectum?"

In fact, v. Gebsattel already knows from the outset that man has a disposition and tendency toward evil, toward sin and toward the nothing, and that the satisfaction of these destructive needs as well as of erotic strivings can bring a "libidinal pleasure." For if v. Gebsattel's anthropology and moral theology do not already presuppose all this, he certainly could not crown his critique of Boss with the anecdote which is given below and even trust it with the key to unlocking the mystery of the sexual perversions. As v. Gesbattel suspects, it stems not by chance from the circle of the last great French pessimist and moralist [Nicola] Chamfort [1741-1974] [182] who committed suicide in 1794. He refers to her as follows: "It concerns a charming, but probably

---

1   Boss's note: M. Heidegger, *Holzwege* [*Off the Beaten Path*], 1954, pp. 86 and 103 [= p. 84].

A. Early Publications Influenced by Martin Heidegger

somehow easily corrupted young lady. In some hot area—let us say Naples—she affords herself enjoyment of a *gelatto*. A sigh escapes her while slurping up the cooling food, but this sigh does not transport her to immediate enjoyment. Instead, her exclamation reveals its real meaning: 'Oh, too bad it's not a peach!' "So," v. Gebsattel concludes, "the coolness giving delicacy lacks something in order to become full enjoyment, something our young miss evidently misses; namely, the sinful impact of its enjoyment, of this moral or, better, immoral element by means of which the sensuous immediacy of inclusiveness would initially be surmounted, were it only that her sigh which showed her sensual enjoyment were what she really relished."[1]

But what if this young lady was not so corrupt and immoral, if she had only been a particularly lively girl? What if a lack of vitality-inhibiting, pseudomoralistic sin preventing guilt would have been to blame for her lack of enjoyment in eating *gelatto*, though that was because she lacked any possibility of overcoming and breaking through such barriers? We know all too well that a lot of bigoted prudish barriers then curtailed the lives of young girls. But with what right then would v. Gebsattel call the desire for a surmounting and breaking out of such bondage a predilection for evil, for destruction and nothingness? Couldn't this girl's wish for "sin" be more reasonably understood as an immediately pleasurable move toward "inclusiveness," toward self-liberation and permission for conventionally forbidden possibilities that belong to its very essence of life, rather than toward "nihilism"?

Boss's text is in response to a critique by Viktor Emil von Gebsattel (1883-1976) published in 1954.[2] Our goal is not to evaluate the discussion but merely to point out references to Heidegger, in this case his 1938 lecture "The Age of the World Picture [Weltbild]" and " Building Dwelling Thinking" from 1951. The theme of the latter is secondary

---

1 Boss's note: von Gebsattel, *loc. cit.*, 220.
2 For a brief introduction to von Gebsattel's "anthropological medicine," see Jos V. M. Welie, "Viktor Emil von Gebsattel on the Doctor-Patient Relationship," in *Theoretical Medicine and Bioethics* **16**(1), 1995, pp. 41-72.

A. Early Publications Influenced by Martin Heidegger

status of symbols in interpreting things which Boss considers when rejecting von Gebsattel's emphasis on the symbolic value of a patient's productions. More important is Heidegger's indictment of anthropology and other secondary sciences such as sociology and psychology. Both Binswanger and von Gebsattel spoke of their approaches as anthropological but here Boss is concerned more with the inherent limitations of what anthropology is supposed to accomplish than with the love of the "humanity" of the patient, which Binswanger and von Gebsattel wanted to bring back into psychotherapy with their emphasis on the existing human being as *anthropos*.

Heidegger's point is that a man-centered interpretation of what is there—where the human being is the alpha and omega of all things—is in no position to ask just what the human being is because it has already decided what man is, namely, a *subiectum* (subject) which is defined by its opposition and separation from *obiecta* (objects). Boss is also concerned in this text to distance himself from the moral implications of von Gebsattel's interpretation, one that Heidegger also eschewed in his analytics of existence. With Nietzsche, existence is *jenseits* (this side of) good and evil. A therapist must also be positioned there, without consideration of what is good or bad about the patient, without evaluation of the other. A tendency toward nihilism in the paraphile is also rejected. As the example illustrates, the girl's gesture (sigh) and comment need not be read as examples of depravity or moral degradation, but instead as deprivation, a "lively" girl's inclination toward fulfillment of life's possibilities. To the offer life holds out for maximal involvement, Boss does not asked "Why?"—as though there were something suspect about such an inclination—but instead "Why not?"

2. *Psychoanalyse und Daseinsanalytik*[1]

In 1957, Boss published *Psychoanalyse und Daseinsanalytik*, which as the title suggests compares psychoanalysis and Heidegger's analytics

---

1   A more thorough comparative study of the original German work and the translation and the fate of what should have been a major influence on psychiatry is in order as a companion to this study. In particular, the notes by the

A. Early Publications Influenced by Martin Heidegger

of existence. In 1963, a book entitled *Psychoanalysis and Daseinsanalysis* was published in a translation by Ludwig Lefebre, a psychotherapist in California who had been Boss's student in Zürich. As already noted, the two books have little to do with each other. As Boss notes in his preface to the English volume, after 1961-1962, when he had lectured in the States, what was to be a translation of *Psychoanalyse und Daseinsanalytik* turned into a very much expanded text, "three times as long as the German original. The enormous differences between the American and the European ways of dealing with such a subject [a comparison of classical psychoanalysis and Heidegger's *Analytik* of *Dasein*] made longer explanations inevitable" (p. v).

A translator's note to the first sentence of *Psychoanalysis and Daseinsanalysis* is the source of much of the confusion surrounding Boss's approach to psychotherapy and had its origin with this volume. I quote the note in full:

> *Daseinsanalysis,* meaning 'analysis of *Dasein,*' is the Anglicized version of the German term *Daseinsanalyse.* Boss uses this term to designate his transformation of psychoanalytic theory and practice, basing his approach on the philosopher Martin Heidegger's *Daseinsanalytik* (which also means 'analysis of *Dasein*') as set forth in Heidegger's *Sein und Zeit*....
>
> *Dasein* is a key term in the work of Heidegger and his followers. Its literal translation is 'to be (*sein*) there (*da*)' and its popular translation is 'existence'. Heidegger uses it in its literal sense, which differs from ordinary German usage. As Heidegger uses it *Dasein* is, in all truth, a new word in the German language. For this reason, and because the only accurate translation—'to be there'—would be too clumsy, I have decided to use the word *Dasein* untranslated in the present book. *Daseinsanalytik*, the term Heidegger uses for his fundamental-ontological analyses of human being, I translate 'analysis of *Dasein*'. [/] The term

---

translator need to be interpreted in detail order to make sense of certain misunderstandings of the project of existential analysis from Binswanger to Boss. See also Andrew J. Mitchell, "Heidegger's Breakdown: Health and Healing under the Care of Dr. V.E. von Gebsattel," in *Research in Phenomenology* 46(1), 2016, pp. 70-97.

A. Early Publications Influenced by Martin Heidegger

Daseinsanalyse was originally introduce by Ludwig Binswanger to characterize his method for investigating psychopathological phenomena and to distinguish this method from Heidegger's ontological analyses, *Daseinsanalytik*. (Although Heidegger provided the starting point for Binswanger's work, the latter has recently stated that he misunderstood Heidegger, adding that he hopes the misunderstanding will be a fruitful one. See L. Binswanger, "Daseinsanalyse und Psychotherapie," in *Acta Psychotherapeutica et Psychosomatica*, Vol. 8, No. 4, 1960, p. 258.)

For clarity I have decided to use 'Daseinsanalysis' and its derivative forms 'Daseinsanalytic' and 'Daseinsanalyst' to designate Boss's approach exclusively. This decision has been facilitated by the fact that Binswanger's method has already been referred to in American publications as 'existential analysis.' See, for example, *Existence*, edited by Rollo May, Ernest Angel, and Henri F. Ellenberger (New York, 1958), which contains two case histories of Binswanger.

The term 'Daseinsanalysis' is not an anglicized version of a German word. In English, nouns are not capitalized. Nor would the possessive in German be carried over in an English word. In psychology, we have preserved words such as Gestalt but they are not part of an artificial compound such as 'Daseinsanalysis'. At best, the term is only a partly anglicized version of a German word. It should have been rendered "analysis of existence" or, following Lefebre's own translation of *Dasein*, "analysis of the to-be-there," whether or not the locution is awkward. Something incomprehensible to most readers in any case is not preferable to a cumbersome expression that prompts reflection. In the end, as we know, Boss himself settled on 'da-seinanalysis'. And yet the construction "to-be-there" is not the only "accurate translation" of *Dasein*. In fact, it is not accurate at all, since in German the particle 'to' is not given with a verb as it is in English (e.g., "to be," "to have," "to write"). With this in mind, an "accurate translation" would be "being there" or "be there." William Richardson's hyphenated term "there-being" (but not capitalized) is probably still the best option when one wants to highlight the elements of the word as Heidegger hears it, in particular the preposition *da*.

A. Early Publications Influenced by Martin Heidegger

Lefebre goes on to say that *Daseinsanalytik* and *Daseinsanalyse* both translate as "analysis of Dasein." More confusion is introduced since we are not consistently reminded in the ensuing text when one or the other word is being translated with the same phrase.

It is true that in "ordinary German usage" *Dasein* denotes existence, but as a *terminus technicus* in the early Heidegger it *also* means existence heard and understood in a certain way, namely, as referring to human beings only. That is the key observation to be made, but one that you have to look for carefully in Lefebre's note. From early on in *Sein und Zeit*, *Dasein* is also always understood to thought in relation to existing (*Existenz*), which Heidegger will relate to the Latin verb *eksistere*.

In Boss's text immediately following the note, we find a sentence in which 'Dasein' and 'existence' are said to be interchangeable. That is not the case. Was this only a matter of reminding us of the difference between the technical usage and the ordinary usage of *Dasein*, or did Boss write a different word for 'existence', for example, *Existenz*? Since this volume is based on a manuscript other than the German original, we have no way of knowing until Boss's papers are available to inspect.

Lefebre adds even more haze by first characterizing Heidegger's *Daseinsanalytik* as the name for "his fundamental-ontological analyses of human being" and only a bit later speaking of the *Daseinsanalytik* as "ontological analyses" (without the "fundamental- "). Also, why the plural ('analyses'), unless it is meant to resonate with -*analyse* (analysis)? Again, referring to Heidegger's project as an analytics (not an analysis) of existence would have been helpful.

Lefebre reflects on Boss's comparison between one form of analysis (psychoanalysis) and another (Daseinsanalysis), but the important terminological distinction to be made is between an analytics of existence (referring to a philosophical endeavor) and an analysis of existence (referring to a psychotherapeutic practice comparable to psychoanalysis as an analysis of the psyche or soul) is not clearly made. The problem may not have been entirely the translator's, however. It may well have been Boss's choice to distance himself from the German book and gain some traction in promoting a new "psychiatric-psychotherapeutic school" (p. 2). In doing so, however, the reader is set up for failing to appreciate the central

A. Early Publications Influenced by Martin Heidegger

point about Heidegger's analytics of existence as a basis for Boss's revision of psychoanalysis, especially in order to differentiate it from the analysis (*Analyse*) carried out in Freud's "procedure," said to be "patterned on certain chemical analyses" with its "aim to dissolve man into his component parts." Heidegger's goal was to delineate the elements of a structure as a whole and not to take it apart as planned to do with his "dismantling" of the history of metaphysics. Boss was clear on this, but the prospective reader of *Psychoanalysis and Daseinsanalysis* is not after reading the first translator's note.

Lefebre's note next acknowledges the origin of the term *Daseinsanalyse* with Ludwig Binswanger as denoting a "method for investigating psychopathological phenomena" (p. 3). Boss's greater interest, however, is in his form of treatment. Binswanger's misunderstanding of Heidegger as having carried out an anthropological investigation is acknowledged, but we are not equipped with the terminology that would keep the two versions of *Daseinsanalyse* apart in the ensuing discussion. To this day, the differences are not clearly apparent to the reader of Boss. Of course, one goal of the present study is to clear the way for a fresh appreciation of Boss's genuinely fresh ideas.

Finally, "for clarity," Lefebre says, he has limited the use of the terms 'Daseinsanalysis', 'Daseinsanalytic', and 'Daseinsanalyst' to Boss's *Daseinsanalyse*. Here again, conventional usage and orthography are not observed. The odd capitalization of an adjective and the name of a practitioner of *Daseinsanalyse* are again not helpful in attaining accuracy and clarity. A practitioner of *Daseinsanalyse* would be, in German, a *Daseinsanalytiker*, a term that might easily be mistaken for something to do with the *Daseinsanalytik*. Lefebre associates Binswanger with his representation in Rollo May's *Existence*, published the year after *Psychoanalyse und Daseinsanalytik*. In his preface, Boss thanks May for his "never-ending help and advice" in preparing *Psychoanalysis and Daseinsanalysis* for publication. We are left with the impression, however, that everyone would have been served better by closer cooperation among the editors, translators, and Boss. Binswanger did not die until 1966 and even he might have been consulted by Boss on the matter.

The book is notable for containing an excerpt from one of Heidegger's letters to the author presumably written sometime before

A. Early Publications Influenced by Martin Heidegger

1963 when the book was published. The passage does not appear in Boss's *Zollikoner Seminare* (1987), however, which contains passages from letters Heidegger letters had written to the author between 1947-1971. What is found in Boss's note is curious for being at variance from the translator's note on one of the terms discussed. Reflecting on how to render *Seyn,* Boss writes that he "had a great many discussions and has exchanged many letters with Heidegger concerning possible English translations for the three terms which are fundamental to Daseinsanalytic thinking…. We reproduce a passage from one of Heidegger's letters verbatim":

> The suggestion to translate (a) *das Seiende* or *Seiendes* as "being" or "particular being," (b) *Seiendheit*, in the sense of the mode of being of a specific species of things or living beings, as "being-ness" (lower case), and (c) *Seyn*, as such, as "*Being-ness*" (capitalized) seems best. To be sure, in the sufficient distinction between (b) and (c) the whole road of my thinking is concealed, insofar as one follows its progression through the essence of metaphysics. It is probably not accidental that the "ontological difference"[1] cannot be adequately stated in either English or French.

Six pages earlier, however, the translator had written: "Following a suggestion by Professor William Bossart of the University of California, I translate *Seiendes* as 'particular being(s)'…. More literal translations of *Seiendes* are 'that which is', actuality', and 'entity'" (p. 31, note). A few questions come to mind. Were Boss and Lefebre not comparing notes and letters? They coincided on 'particular being', but for different words. *Das Seiende* covers the singular for 'entity', 'essent', 'being', or 'particular being', but inflected it can also refer to "all of what is there."

Heidegger's understanding of English would not have been authoritative, however. Indeed, in his letter to Boss of August 10, 1960, he wrote in response to a request to accompany Boss to the States to teach: "*One* major difficulty is my very poor command of English. I

---

1 Here Lefebre interpolates "[i.e., the distinction between (b) [*Seiendheit*] and (c) [*Seyn*]]."

A. Early Publications Influenced by Martin Heidegger

cannot speak the language at all and can barely understand spoken English."[1] Yet Boss seems to rely on it with respect to how to translate Heidegger's neologism. I am not aware that *Seyn* has been translated anywhere else as 'Being-ness', in contrast with 'being-ness' (for *Seiendheit*) as referring to "the mode of being of a specific species of things or living beings." Perhaps we should question the translation of the letter by Lefebre.

Overall, then, there should be much to feel uneasy about when looking back to *Psychoanalysis and Daseinsanalysis*, especially since it was most clinical psychologists' introduction to the new form of psychoanalysis Boss was presenting. At the least, it leaves one befuddled about Heidegger's contribution, both theoretical and personal. Following the "Outline of Analysis of *Dasein*" (Chapter 2), which is intended to be read as a summary of Heidegger's analytics of existence, Boss writes (p. 49) that he had "Martin Heidegger's untiring personal help in compiling the foregoing summary." I wonder, however, whether Heidegger would have approved of it as translated.

Although Lefebre is the only translator named on the title page and in standard bibliographic sources, in fact much of the case material (about 60 pages of all 285 pages of the book) was translated by Elsa Lehman, MD (chapters 1, 7, 11 and 20) and Mary-Hottinger Mackie (chapter 11, as co-translator with Lehman). Translational discrepancies between their work and Lefebre's bear examination.[2]

A quick look at two reviews of the book provides varying perspectives on the influence of the analytics of existence on existential analysis. *Psychoanalysis and Daseinsanalysis* was discussed in the *Review of Metaphysics*[3] and *The Psychoanalytic*

---

1 ZS 319-320 / ZO 255. He adds, on translation: "Through translation everything gets changed and becomes wearisome. My way of thinking and the phenomenological approach will probably still be strange over there." And so it is.
2 Elsa Lehman, MD, was a New York psychiatrist who taught at the Cornell University—New York Hospital School of Nursing. Mary Hottinger-Mackie was a translator who taught English at the University of Zürich.
3 Peter A. Bertocci, "Existential Phenomenology and Psychoanalysis," in *The Review of Metaphysics* 18(4), 1965, 690-720. This "critical study" looks at four "studies in psychopathology": Herbert Fingarette (a philosopher), *The Self in Transformation*; Karl Jaspers', *General Psychopathology*; Ludwig Binswanger, *Being-in-the-World*; and Boss's *Psychoanalysis and Daseinsanalysis*. He takes for granted that

A. Early Publications Influenced by Martin Heidegger

Review.[1] It is enough for our purposes to point out that, at least for one philosopher familiar with and open to the Continental tradition, the distinction between *Daseinsanalyse* as a treatment modality and Heidegger's *Daseinsanalytik* was clear (pp. 698-699). Bertocci's interest in several approaches to psychopathology raises the question whether the uniqueness of existential analysis ultimately lies in minimizing considerations of psychopathology in favor of recognizing the challenge to each of us of inevitabilities of existing. Instead of encounter framed by considerations of causality, interest in the past, and interventional involvement with the other, all of which are grounded in the medical model and ask the question "Why?," encounter between one existence and another based on a Heidegger's analytics of existence abandons all of that and leads to Boss's famous "Why not?," which is non-interventional and concentrates on the present of the other. This will occupy us in the concluding part of the present study.

For the psychoanalyst, who is firmly committed to categories of psychopathology, in the context of "the 'existentialism' business," says Curry, Boss's attempt "to demonstrate how *Daseinsanalysis* fits into the psychoanalytic model" is welcomed, especially for the case study that describes "a clinical picture so moving in its drama, so compelling in its humanness, that I know of nothing—save in literature—that compares." This is high praise, especially given the common impression among analysts about the literary quality of Freud's case histories. He is also appreciative of the book's "most penetrating re-evaluation of the psychoanalytic 'doctrine of neurosis.'"

The reviewer recognizes that, as based on his theoretical model, what Freud *said* he did and others should do did not always correspond to what he actually *did*. The same probably held for Boss. The central issue is whether an existential analysis fully realized is not precluded by the clinical setting, especially in a time when psychotherapy

---

> Heidegger's *Dasein* is a familiar enough notion, even though *Being and Time* had been published only the year before the four volumes under consideration were published. At one point, however, he glosses the term with "life-being" (p. 697). In the discussion of Binswanger, he has *Dasein* as both neuter and gendered: "Each Dasein, dealing with its existential anxieties, construes *his life-space* in relation to others" (p. 697).

1 Andrew E. Curry, review in *Psychoanalytic Review* **51B**(2), 1964, 159-160.

A. Early Publications Influenced by Martin Heidegger

is construed as a service sold by healthcare providers. Curry seems to understand the phenomenological view of practice Boss presents: "Though the space of activity is a small office, that activity, in a deeper sense, stretches out toward a horizon which exceeds our vision . . .. If our psychotherapeutic endeavors do not aim toward that horizon then our commitment to the profession is shallow indeed" (pp. 159-160).

My claim in the end will be that existential analysis as based on Heidegger's analytics of existence, transcends the requirements of the clinical setting and that although he could not take the step out of that setting, Boss made it possible for others to do so.

B. The Two Dream Books

The two dream books—1953 and 1975—precede and follow the period of the Zollikon seminars. The translations—1958 and 1977—suffer in many places from the same sort of problems we have already seen, though to a less extent in the first, *The Analysis of Dreams*.[1] There we read, for example, of both "existentialist analysis" and "existential analysis" (pp. 10, 118). On the other hand, the magic spell of the word '*Dasein*' was broken by the translator, Arnold J. Pomerans,[2] only to reappear, however, with Stephen Conway's translation of the second dream book, "*I dreamt last night*..." (e.g., pp. 41, 51).[3] There we find peculiar sentences such as: "The existence, or *Da-sein*, which is the common matrix of both waking and dreaming reveals itself to an unbiased observer as an 'ecstatic' opening up of that clearance which we call 'world'" (p. 185).

In the second dream book, Boss consistently writes *Da-sein* (hyphenated). He also speaks of both *Existenz* and *Da-sein*, and it is not always made clear to the reader when one or the other is translated with 'existence'. Stephen Conway went on to work with Anne Cleaves on the translation of the *Grundriß der Medizin und der Psychologie* published in 1977.[4]

---

1 Full bibliographic information is found in my *An International Bibliography of the Writings of Medard Boss (1929-2003)* below.
2 Arnold J. Pomerans was a well-known and accomplished German-born British translator who also translated Freud, Piaget and Huizinga.
3 Stephen Conway also translated Klaus Theweleit's *Männerfantasien* (two volumes, 1977-1978), psychoanalytic studies of Weimar Republic males.
4 Yarrow Anne Cleaves, who assisted Conway, was an English major at Mt. Holyoke College (class of '65) and would have been in her early thirties when working with Conway.

B. The Two Dream Books

1. *The Analysis of Dreams*

In the foreword of the first dream book by E. B. Strauss, then president of the British Psychological Society, Boss is introduced as a "phenomenological psychiatrist," and both an "existentialist psychotherapist" and a "[psycho]analytical psychotherapist" (p. 7). Boss speaks of himself as a "psycho-analytical therapist" and simply a "psychotherapist" with a background of "training in classical psycho-analytical theory and practice" (p.9). Boss writes that his revision of the Freudian (and Jungian) approaches to dream interpretation was "owing to my contact with the existentialist analytical approach of Martin Heidegger. Stimulated by the work of Ludwig Binswanger, I have made a thorough study of Heidegger's published, and even of some of his unpublished, writings, and then benefitted from Heidegger's unstinting readiness for direct discussion. Whether I have the mind for the strict detail demanded by existentialist analysis and its discussion, can only be decided by this work" (p. 10).

The preface makes it clear that long before the seminars during the first five years of their acquaintance, Boss was already on intimate terms with Heidegger. In a letter of January 26, 1952, Heidegger alludes to his familiarity with Boss's work on his first dream book. It seems that Heidegger related some of his own dreams to Boss during one of their families' vacations together: "Hopefully, you were in a state of creative alertness for the 'dreams' during the vacations. I always think that the work could be of great and fundamental importance and could turn all therapy away from 'psychology.'"[1]

Later that year (August 2, 1952), Heidegger wrote about material he had received from Boss in a letter:

> The added section is clear and correct (introduction to the book by Medard Boss, *Der Traum und seine Auslegung* [1953]). In the final paragraph, an addendum would be suitable. It would simply sharpen what you already state and what pervades the whole

---

[1] ZS 305 / ZO 242. The translators of the English edition mistake the second edition of *Der Traum und seine Auslegung* (1974) for the second edition of Boss's second dream (1991) (ZO 245, note).

B. The Two Dream Books

work: not to give a causal explanation and derivation of the dreams, but to let the dreams themselves tell their own stories by what they say and reveal in their orientation toward the world. Dreams are not symptoms and consequences of something hidden lying behind [them], but they themselves are in what they show and *only* this. Only with *this* does their essence become worthy of questioning.

My lecture course came to a good close. I still have to add a very difficult passage, which I omitted. Then I will proceed with the other thing. Hopefully, the start will be successful. Last night, the examination dream promptly reappeared.[1]

The translators omit a very important note to the excerpt by Boss. It has been mentioned in biographical comments on Heidegger, but it is especially notable for its omission here in connection with the first dream book. It is Heidegger's reminder to Boss of his recurring examination dream, with which Boss was evidently familiar:

As Martin Heidegger has expressed himself, this refers to the only dream he remembers which has constantly recurred since his youth, albeit for the most part at greater intervals. In this dream situation, he again and again experiences himself in nearly the same way as he was in high school and is examined by the same professors who at that time in waking life examined him [to qualify] for graduation. There is eventually enough of this recurring dream when it is possible for him to experience being in the light of the event and in wakeful thinking, thus attaining its 'fruition.'"[2]

---

1 ZS 307-308 / ZO 245. Heidegger is referring to the preface (*Vorwort*), not the introduction (*Einleitung*), from which we have quoted above.

2 ZS 308, note 2. "Bezieht sich auf den wie Martin Heidegger sich ausdrükte einzigen, aber seit seiner Jugend ständig, wenn auch meist in größeren Abständen wiederkehrenden Traum, an den er sich erinnert. In diesen Traumzuständen erfährt er sich immer wieder in ganz ähnlicher Art im Gymnasium und wird von den gleichen Professoren geprüft, die ihn seinerzeit auch im Arbitur seines Wachlebens prüften. Endgültig war es mit diesem stereotypen Traum vorbei, als er im wachen Denken *Sein* im Lichte des Ereignisses zu erfahren vermochte,

B. The Two Dream Books

One wonders what Boss said to Heidegger about this dream, equivalent to Freud's dream of "Irma's injection," on "the experience of being in the light of the event." Is this not the very heart of Heidegger's thought?

It remains to point out a few places in the first dream book that seem to be of major importance to our theme. Here he makes the radical assertion that "existential analysis as such is indifferent both to psychotherapeutic techniques and to practical consequences and aims" (p. 119). All the same, in the following paragraphs, which refer explicitly to Heidegger, he speaks of the existential analytical psychotherapist "keeping as closely as possible to Freud's practical indications" and of "the deeper and existential meaning of Freud's technical rules" (pp. 119-120). Here he refers to the fundamental rule, free association, "evenly suspended [hovering] attention," and use of the couch. He also refers to interpretation and the analysis of resistance and transference. It is important to recall, however, that by the time of his very important paper "Encounter in Psychotherapy" (1964), Boss had realized that transference was an indefensible concept.[1] This important section of the book ends with a summary of Boss's view of the dream (p. 122). Heidegger's direct influence is mentioned again on several occasions (pp. 183, 194 ff.), where the reader must again be cautious about the distinction Heidegger makes between *Dasein* and *Existenz* and when one or the other term is being translated as 'existence'.

2. "I dreamt last night..."

Although published only a year before Heidegger's death, the second dream book was under discussion by Heidegger and Boss in 1972 (see ZS 288-291 / ZO 228-231, and 340, note 1). In it, Heidegger's influence is acknowledged (pp. xv, 46, 182, 186-187), but once again in many places the reader is uncertain about just what Heidegger's words were. Key terms are sometimes translated and other times not. In general, the

---

damit dessen 'Reife' erlangend." See also the March 2, 1972, conversation—ZS 289 / ZO 229—in which the dream is mentioned.

[1] "Begegnung in der Psychotherapie," in *Psychotherapy and Psychosomatics* **13**(5), 1965, pp. 332-341.

B. The Two Dream Books

volume was not carefully edited. Again, Boss certainly deserved better. It probably did not help the psychiatrists, "sociologists, educators, psychotherapists, and religious practitioners" for whom it was written as "a simple exercise book" (p. xxi) for practitioners of dream interpretation to find words glossed with the original German, especially when presenting Heidegger's terminology (e.g., p. 187). Odd constructions such as *Daseins*-analysis and *Daseins*-analyst, *Dasein* or *Da-sein* confront the reader unprepared to understand their sense. The word *Dasein* seems just to drop in (p. 31) following talk of "human existence," unannounced except in the chapter title ("The Phenomenological or *Daseins*-analytic Understanding of Dreams") in which it appears.

C. The *magnum opus*: Existential Foundations of Medicine and Psychology

Boss's *Outline of Medicine and Psychology: Approaches to Phenomenological Physiology, Psychology, Pathology and Therapy, and an Existential Preventative Medicine*—as I would translate the volume's full title—is a textbook for physicians.[1] It was not intended to be beyond the reach and grasp of those who lacked medical training, however. Few doctors, including psychiatrists, living today have heard of this book. Perhaps that is fortuitous for the profession, since the *Grundriß* is among only a few works that might serve as a radical re-envisioning of the profession. It is also a possible starting point of a declaration of independence of psychotherapy from the medical model. Might psychiatry "cede" from medicine? Not likely, but some

---

1   The book is known, of course, as *Existential Foundations of Medicine and Psychology*, edited by Paul J. Stern and, I surmise, Boss himself (New York: Jason Aronson, 1979) [= EF]. The translation is based on Boss's *Grundriß der Medizin und der Psychologie: Ansätze zu einer phänomenologischen Physiologie, Psychologie, Pathologie und Therapie und zu einer daseinsgemäßen Präventiv-Medizin* (Hans Huber, 2nd enlarged edition 1975) [= GM]. The subtitle, which explicitly refers to psychology, was not retained for the English translation and remained the same as in the first edition (1971) of the book. In 1994, the second edition was reissued with a preface by the author's widow, Marianne Boss-Linsmayer. It has also been translated into Slovak (1985) and Czech (1992).

C. *The* magnum opus

have suggested that psychiatry is a discipline that came into being in a particular historical context and is about to disappear, much as psychosomatics disappeared when several years ago consultation-liaison psychiatry came into being.[1]

Heidegger carefully examined the manuscript of the *Grundriß*, as he had the first dream book, but he also played a major role in its genesis and evolution. Heidegger "is responsible for this attempt to lay out a foundation for medicine [and psychology]" (EF xxiii). Two decades later, echoing the addendum to the preface to the dream book, Boss is more expansive. The book, he writes, "reflects the countless conversations in which I was privileged to participate over two decades of friendship. For the past fifteen years, Heidegger has held two or three seminars each semester for the benefit of medical students, including mine. The discussions coming out of these 'Zollikon Seminars' also figure significantly in this work. More important, though, is the fact that this work actually evolved under Heidegger's watchful eye. There is not one section of 'philosophical' import which was denied his generous criticism" (EF xxiii–xxiv).

The first edition of the book was published as *Grundriß der Medizin* (1971). In the preface to the second, "enlarged" edition (1975), Boss wrote: "The title of the first edition, as it turned out, failed to express the author's original intent; it seemed to indicate that the book could be understood only by physicians. I had assumed with too much haste that everyone would recognize a foundation of medicine based on human nature as, necessarily, a foundation of psychology and sociology as well" (p. xxv). And so it became the *Grundriß der Medizin und der Psychologie*.

The book consists of three parts: an outline of medicine as currently understood, the sketch of a contrasting human [*menschengerecht*] medicine, and approaches to an existentially informed [*daseinsgemäße*] pathology (etiology, pathogenesis, and phenomenology of being ill [*Krank-sein*]). In a fourth part Boss offers some notes [*Hinweise*] on an existentially informed therapy [*daseinsgemäße Therapie*] and an

---

1 See my article "Medicine and Dasein-therapy. Medard Boss and the Beginnings of a Human Therapeutics," in *Free Associations. Psychoanalysis and Culture, Media, Groups, Politics* **#46**, September 2019, pp. 108-135.

C. The magnum opus

approach to preventative medicine from an existential perspective "in modern industrial society."

The English translation by Stephen Conway and Anne Cleaves, entitled *Existential Foundations of Medicine and Psychology*, was supplied with an introduction by Paul J. Stern. It was said to be a "somewhat abridged" (p. xvii) version of the second German edition. In fact, it was extensively reduced. The second edition of the *Grundriß* runs to about 154,000 words; the translation is 28,000 words shy of that. In addition, in Part One of the translation there has also been a rearrangement of sections in order to begin the book with Boss's *Testfall* (test case), "Regula Zürcher," which appears after the introductory material found in Boss's original text. As mentioned, the subtitle has been omitted. In it, Boss had named (in order) physiology, pathology, psychology, therapy and, in general, an existentially-informed [*daseinsgemäßig*] approach to preventive medicine to which the author proposes to provide approaches [*Ansätze*]. Apart from *psychology* all of the areas mentioned belong to medicine. This raises the question of how Boss saw the relation between academic psychology and psychiatry. *Therapy* refers throughout to both a form of medical treatment and psychoanalysis as a modality of psychotherapy.

His English-speaking readers are reminded that any sort of ground plan for medical practice "based on human nature" must also be a ground plan for psychology, academic and applied, *and* sociology. This is an interesting expansion that points to the final chapter of Boss's book, which is given as an "Afterword" in the English version.

An editor is referred to (e.g., p. xxxi), but none is named in the credits. Since translators' notes are acknowledged differently, we might assume the editor was Boss himself, whose English was excellent, or Paul Stern, or that they shared in the work of editing. By the time Boss realized the book should be translated into English, probably sometime before the 1975 German edition was prepared (the preface to that edition is dated "Spring 1974"), and as he worked out translation and editorial responsibilities with Stern, Conway, Cleaves and Jason Aronson, Boss likely realized that American readers might be overwhelmed by the long theoretical preliminaries found in his original text and he therefore condensed it. Boss probably also realized that people outside of medicine would be attracted by the word

C. *The* magnum opus

'existential' in the title, linking his book with the tradition of "existential psychology and psychiatry" that had developed in the 1960s. Rollo May's anthology *Existence* (1958) had only recently brought European psychology and psychiatry (especially Ludwig Binswanger, Erwin Straus and Viktor von Gebsattel) to the attention of American readers. Associations were also made with the tradition of "humanistic psychology" that originated as the "Third Force" of American psychology beginning with Gordon Allport and Carl Rogers.

D. The Zollikon Seminars

We come now to the centerpiece of our study, that series of meetings with psychiatrists and others dominated by the presence of Martin Heidegger that Boss hosted at his home.

1. Zollikon Seminars: Protocols–Conversations–Letters

In Spring 1987, Medard Boss edited for publication *Zollikoner Seminare. Protokolle—Gespräche—Briefe* by his mentor and friend, Martin Heidegger.[1] Thirty years later, the same publisher issued Heidegger's *Zollikoner Seminare* as Volume 89 (2018) of Heidegger's *Complete Edition [Gesamtausgabe]*, edited by Peter Trawny.[2] Heidegger's numerous notes and annotations now available are a rich source of ideas that that may yet rescue therapy [*Therapie*] from the medical model. A comparison of the editions will provide an opportunity to better understand where Boss was unable to follow his mentor in influencing physicians in their approach to the care of other human beings. It will also afford us an opportunity to note some of Heidegger's observations on a variety of topics.

---

1 Martin Heidegger, *Zollikoner Seminare. Protokolle—Gespräche—Briefe* (Frankfurt: Klostermann, 1987; ²1994; ³2006)—edited, of course, by Medard Boss (XXXII + 880 pp.) [= *ZS*].
2 Martin Heidegger, *Zollikoner Seminare* (Frankfurt: Klostermann, 2018)—edited by Peter Trawny (XXVIII + 369 pp.) [= *GA*].

D. The Zollikon Seminars

The Boss edition was translated into English in 2001.[1] Apart from several books (reviewed above) and several papers published by Boss, until now the minutes of the seminars prepared by Boss, supplemented by records of selected conversations with Heidegger (from 1961 to 1972), and 110 excerpts of Heidegger's letters to Boss (from 1947 to 1971), have been the only source of our understanding the development of that form of psychoanalysis known as *Daseinsanalyse*.

Given its length, a translation of *GA 89* is not likely to appear for a very long time, but it is essential that as we become familiar with its contents now. It is crucial that Heidegger scholars waste no time in gleaning from what is found in the pages of *GA 89* what Heidegger provided for practitioners of therapy that might lead to a revival of the calling on a footing that is not tethered to the medical model. I now provide only a guide for doing that but soon hope to publish a selection of Heidegger's notes that are most provocative and not already known to us from the Boss edition of the Zollikon seminars.

As in so many other areas—philosophy, art, technology and the media, ecology—Heidegger's remarkable rethinking (following Kant) of the question "What is man?" will turn out to be crucial for those who

---

1 Martin Heidegger, *Zollikon Seminars. Protocols—Conversations—Letters* (Medard Boss, ed.) (Evanston: Northwestern University Press, 2001), translated by Richard Askay and Franz Mayr (xxxiii + 360 pp.) [= *TR*]. Ten years later one of the translators, Richard Askay, published *Of Philosophers and Madmen. A Disclosure of Martin Heidegger, Medard Boss, and Sigmund Freud* (New York: Rodopi, 2011). This book begins with a "play," "Of Philosophers and Madmen" (modeled on the title of John Steinbeck's *Of Mice and* Men), in which Heidegger is portrayed as having suffered from a psychological disorder for which he received inpatient medical treatment by Boss and in the course of which Sigmund Freud's presence is imagined. Several essays complement the play. Two earlier publications of excerpts from ZS appeared as Martin Heidegger, "Martin Heidegger's Zollikon Seminars," in *The Review of Existential Psychology and Psychiatry* (Pittsburgh) 16 (1-3), 1978-79, pp. 7-20, translated by Brian Kenny (reprinted as Keith Hoeller (ed.), *Heidegger and Psychology* (1988) Seattle: Review of Existential Psychology and Psychiatry, pp. 7-20), and Martin Heidegger, "On Adequate Understanding of Daseinsanalysis" and "Marginalia an Phenomenology, Transcendence and Care," in *The Humanistic Psychologist* **16**(1), 1988, pp. 75-98 and 218-223, translated by Michael Eldred (excerpts corresponding to pp. 115-116, 120-121, 188-191, 203, 204-205, 205-206, 207, 227-228 and 191-194 of the *ZS*).

D. The Zollikon Seminars

are called to the highly unusual work of therapy.[1] Given what is found in the Trawny edition of the Zollikon seminars, self-examination by psychiatrists and psychoanalysts and others who dabble in psychotherapy in the tradition of *Daseinanalyse* is *de rigeur*.

I have set myself three tasks: first, to familiarize potential readers of the new edition of the seminars with the background of the GA edition as described by its editor in his postscript to GA 89; second, to provide the materials necessary for a detailed comparison of the two editions of the seminars and raise some questions about discrepancies between them; and, third, discuss several examples of Heidegger's insights found in the new edition that are especially relevant to a new beginning for therapy.

Since another major element of the story of the development of Boss's *Daseinsanalyse* was his travels in India as a visiting teacher, physician and seeker, I will go on to have a look at his "India book." I conclude with a brief outline of what "dasein-therapy" might look like.

2. The Two Editions of the *Zollikoner Seminare*

We now have two quite different editions of the Heidegger seminars held in Switzerland from 1959 to 1969. Quite a lot is known about the Boss edition, especially its uniqueness among the other volumes of the *Complete Edition* of Heidegger's writings. Some details about this are provided later by way of reminder. The Trawny edition is so new that it has not been reviewed in any English publication. This contribution may, in part, serve that purpose.

---

[1] For some history of and speculation about the future of what Freud called one of the three "impossible callings" readers may have a look at my publications on what I have for the time being decided to call *dasein-therapy* or simply *therapy* and, in particular, the central place of Medard Boss in the story. See *After Psychotherapy* (New York: ENI Press, 2016).

D. The Zollikon Seminars

a. The Background of the Gesamtausgabe Edition of Zollikoner Seminare

Following is a translation of Peter Trawny's "Editor's Postscript" to *Zollikoner Seminare* (2018).[1] In general, I have rendered Trawny's usages in his discussion of the preparation of GA 89 as follows: *Augzeichnung[en]* → note(s); *Fußnote[n]* → footnote[s]; *Notate* → notes (used once); *Notiz[en]* → notation[s] or note[s]; *Protokoll[en]* → minutes; *Seminar* → seminar. The singular 'seminar' usually refers to a pair of meetings during a week-long visit Heidegger made to Boss's home, where most of the seminars were held. In his edition, Boss published one set of minutes (*Protokoll*) for a week's meetings.

The footnotes are Trawny's as they are found in the *Nachwort*. I have added only three comments, but I have also added in square brackets [1] the dates of people referred to in the postscript mentioned by Heidegger when I could determine them, [2] German words in the original when the usage might be unclear from the context, [3] and an occasional interpolation to make Trawny's sense clearer to the reader. Trawny is a formidable scholar and this volume is an exceptional addition to the material in Part IV of the *Complete Edition*. Appendix A displays in rough outline the layout of the two German editions and the English translation, which is based on the Boss edition.

---

[871] The present Volume 89 of the *Complete Edition* contains all the notes for the thirteen seminars that Martin Heidegger [1889-1976] held in collaboration with the Swiss psychoanalyst Medard Boss [1903-1990] between November 1959 and March 1969, first in the so-called Burghölzli, the Psychiatric Hospital of the University of Zürich, then hosted at Boss's home in Zollikon, a community on the northeastern shore of Lake Zürich in the canton of Zürich. Because the seminars most often took place in Zollikon, Boss's edition of the

---

1 "Nachwort der Herausgebers" (*ZS*, pp. 871-880). Since, unlike Boss's books, it is readily available, I have not included the complete German text. I have been liberal in providing Trawny's original German words, especially when this bears on our project of keeping the sense of key terms clear.

D. The Zollikon Seminars

seminars has been called the "Zollikon seminars" since first published in 1987.[1]

Boss invited already established and still aspiring psychiatrists and psychologists to the seminars. Their influence on the development of psychiatry in Switzerland can be seen to this day.[2] One of Heidegger's documents in the present edition [February 3, 1960, GA 60-61] includes a list of the participants, which conveys the historical dimension of the seminars. A copy of the list and the naming of living persons associated with it were discussed with them.

The present edition coincides in part with that of Boss but includes not only Heidegger's elaborate lecture and seminar notes [*Aufzeichnungen*][3] as well as the minutes [*Protokollen*][4] of the seminar sessions,

---

1 [Translator's comment: As explained above, Trawny uses the singular *Seminar* when referring to pairs of sessions on different days of a given week when Heidegger visited Switzerland to work with Boss and his colleagues. The exceptions are the two Burghölzli sessions, one each in 1959 and 1960, and the conversations with Boss in Taormina, which Trawny refers to as the *third* seminar and designates as the *first* set of recorded minutes. Zürich is a canton of Switzerland or the Swiss Confederacy. Much like a state in the USA, each of the 28 cantons is comprised of a number of districts or *Bezirke*, comparable to our counties. One of the twelve districts of canton Zürich is Meilen and one of its eleven municipalities is Zollikon. In one sense, then, Zollikon is part of Zürich (the canton), but the municipality of Zürich is its own demographic entity.]
2 [Translator's comment: Ania Padrutt (2003). "Bahnhofstraße, Zollikon—Erfahrung in den Zollikoner Seminaren," in Manfred Riedel, Harald Seubert and Hanspeter Padrutt (eds.), *Zwischen Philosophie, Medizin und Psychologie. Heidegger im Dialog mit Medard Boss* (Köln: Böhlau Verlag, 2003), pp. 269-275.]
3 According to Medard Boss, the series of seminars began on September 8, 1959, with a "Lecture by Martin Heidegger in the Great Lecture Hall" XII of the Burghölzli. I am not familiar with the manuscript of this lecture. It cannot be ruled out, however, that Boss has merely used a misleading expression and it was only an introductory comment. Cf. Martin Heidegger, *Zollikoner Seminare. Protokolle—Zwiegespräche—Briefe* (Medard Boss, ed.) (Frankfurt: Vittorio Klostermann, 20063), p. XIII. [Translator's comment: It is interesting that beginning with the second edition (1994), four years after Boss's death, the publisher altered the title. Instead of *Gespräche* (conversations), we find the more formal *Zwiegespräche* (dialogues). Boss had used the term in the subtitle of the second part of his edition, but not in the title. This title was continued with the subsequent edition of 2006 which expanded to include an index. Peter Trawny will refer to the third edition.]
4 Only the first recorded seminar minutes of July 6 and 9, 1964, were prepared by "Miss Dr. med. Erna Hoch [1920-2003]".

D. The Zollikon Seminars

most of which were prepared by Boss himself, but also all the notations [Notizen] Heidegger made in preparation for the seminars and in their thematic sphere. To that thematic [872] sphere belong not only the well-known recorded conversations [Gespräche] between Boss and Heidegger, but also Heidegger's notes about those conversations. Not included were those taken down by Boss and later passed on in the second part of his edition of the "Zollikon seminars" published as "Conversations" (with the exception of the "Conversations with Martin Heidegger in Taormina, Sicily, from April 24 to May 6, 1963") as well excerpts of Heidegger's letters to Boss (in the third part [of Boss's edition]).

The drawing reproduced by Boss, which Heidegger "had drawn on the blackboard of the lecture hall by hand with chalk," was also not included. Heidegger's (according to Boss) "written" note [Notiz] related to it was not available to me and is therefore not included in the present volume.[1]

In addition to Ludwig Binswanger [1881-1966], after a post-war preoccupation with Heidegger's thought Medard Boss developed so-called "existential analysis [Daseinsanalyse]." It is supposed to be an alternative to Sigmund Freud's [1856-1939] "psychoanalysis [Psychoanalyse]." For working out this alternative, the "Zollikon seminars" provided indispensable preparation. To this day, they are still considered to be a founding document [Gründungsdokument] of "existential analysis" as practiced.

In a letter of August 24, 1966, Heidegger writes: "[. . .] I am pleased that the work is moving forward. The seminar minutes are there for you to ensure they are *put to use* and continue to have an effect on science, something that we ourselves alone cannot do."[2] In this respect, the new edition of the *Zollikon Seminars* is intended to place at our disposal more and also different material for work [Arbeitsmaterial].

*

---

1 On inquiring, I was kindly informed that the literary remains [Nachlaß] of Medard Boss are held by the Zürich Zentralbibliothek [City Library], but that (consisting mainly of patient reports) they are not open for "reasons of archival law."
2 Heidegger, *Zollikoner Seminare, op. cit.*, p. 347.

D. The Zollikon Seminars

The following manuscripts housed in the Deutsches Literaturarchiv Marbach were incorporated into Volume 89 of the *Complete Edition* of Heidegger's writings. The sequence of the naming of the manuscripts corresponds to their appearance in the volume:

[873] B 56, 6 Zürich Seminar. Burghölzli, November 1959 (20 sheets of paper)
B 56, 6 Burghölzli, February 3, 1960 (14 sheets of paper)
B 56,6 [Notes of the Burghölzli Seminar] (20 sheets of paper)
B 56, 6 Subjectivity, Consciousness and There-being [*Da-sein*] (March 1960) (31 sheets of paper)
B 59, 3 Sicily. Conversations with Medard Boss, April 23 to May 4, 1963 (27 sheets of paper) with [a] record of conversations with Prof. Martin Heidegger in Taormina, Sicily, from April 24 to May 6, 1963 (18 sheets of paper)
B 74,1 Seminar in connection with the paper "Kant's Thesis about Being" (37 sheets of paper) with minutes from July 6 and 9, 1964 (9 sheets of paper)
B 58,8 Causality and Motivation. Foundations (23 sheets of paper)
D 1,5 [July 9, 1964] (5 sheets of paper)
B 32, 7 The Essence of Contemporary Natural Science and Reflection on the Phenomenon (November 2, 1964) (10 sheets of paper)
B 32,7 Physics (19 sheets of paper)
B 32,7 Nature und "Causality" (5 sheets of paper)
B 32, 7 The Nearby (12 sheets of paper)
B 71 The Question Concerning Time I. January 18 and 21, 1965 (81 sheets of paper)
B 32, 8 T[emporality]. Boss Seminar, March 10, 1965, and On the Interpretation of Visualization. Seminar, March 12, 1965 (44 sheets of paper)
B 71 March Seminar (1965) (13 sheets of paper)
B 71 The Question Concerning Time II (266 sheets of paper)
C 2, 10 Corporeality and Space (55 sheets of paper)
C2, 11a The Spatiality of Existence and Corporeality (3 sheets of paper)
C2, 11b Space and Corporeality (7 sheets of paper)
C2, 11c Place and Space (1 sheet of paper)
C2, 11d Touch (4 sheets of paper)
C22, 3b Recollection and Memory (17 sheets of paper)

D. The Zollikon Seminars

B 58, 8 Corporeality and Situatedness. See *BaT* [*Being and Time*], § 28 ff. (9 sheets of paper)
B 32, 7 Seminar of July 6 and 8, 1965 (96 sheets of paper)
B 32, 8 [On Technology] (20 sheets of paper)
B 58, 8 [Togetherness and Coexistence] (10 sheets of paper)
B 58, 8 Being-in-the-world. I—Thou. "Conversation" (32 sheets of paper)
B 58, 8 Analytics of Existence. Existential Analysis (Seminar, November 1965) (33 sheets of paper)
B 58, 8 Seminar, March 1 and 3, 1966 (38 sheets of paper)
C 2, 1 Consciousness and Existence (March 1969) (29 sheets of paper)
Yellow Portfolio 15 [the minutes with handwritten notations] (74 sheets of paper)[1]

[874] The character and format of the manuscripts differ. Sometimes, for example, such as those for March 10 and 12, 1965 (B 32, 8), Heidegger has precisely formulated them on DIN A5 sheets of paper in black ink underlined in places in red[2] for their oral presentation (similar to the notes for July 6 and 8, 1965, B 32, 7). Other notes, such as those from the conversations with Boss (B 59, 3), were written in pencil and are sometimes very difficult to decipher.

Many sheets [*Zettel*] from the array of manuscripts are fragmentary, preparatory and suggestive in character. In addition, they often give only extracts [*Ekzerpte*]. Heidegger has taken note of, copied out in part, and sometimes commented on academic publications such as Elisabeth Ströker's [1928-2000] *Philosophische Untersuchungen zum Raum* (Frankfurt: Vittorio Klostermann, 1965) and Michael Theunissen's [1932-2015] *Der Andere. Studien zur Sozialontologie der Gegenwart* (Berlin: Walter de Gruyter, 1965). But important new publications on cybernetics such as Norbert Wiener's [1894-1964] *Mensch und Menschmaschine. Kybernetik und Gesellschaft* (Frankfurt: Metzner,

---

1 The titles are the headings given by Heidegger. Titles placed in square brackets were added by me. The upper case letters B, C and D represent an outline of the manuscripts in the form of a list of Heidegger manuscripts which Hermann Heidegger in collaboration with Friedrich-Wilhelm von Herrmann produced during many years of archival work at the German literary archive in Marbach am Neckar.
2 These are not reproduced in my transcription because it would be difficult to separate them in print from the actual underlinings.

D. The Zollikon Seminars

1952) are also noted by him. I have included these and other such references in the present volume. They are found at the places in the volume where they were inserted in the manuscripts.

The question of whether something fragmentary, even marginal, which does not directly belong to the theme should be published in the *Complete Edition* can be answered in different ways. The few notes by Heidegger on the layout [*Gestaltung*] of the manuscript-based [*letzter Hand*] *Complete Edition* leave a great deal of leeway for answering it.[1]

For me, the fact that Heidegger kept and ordered the notes [875] is a sign of his interest in passing them on to posterity. Heidegger is a thinker who is consumed by the power of the single word. Thus even a fragmentary note is a trace [*Spur*] of his thinking.

*

The structure of the volume follows a chronological reconstruction of the sequence of the seminars by Friedrich-Wilhelm von Herrmann [b. 1934]. The arrangement of the manuscripts according to this structure was not always an easy task. In particular, the enormous number of notes was at times the most difficult thing [to deal with].

Only a few notes are available from the "Zürich seminar" of November 1959. But they already document problems Heidegger had to face during all meetings with participants in the seminars. The philosopher had to move about in "*different languages*," that of "*scientific medical practice* [*wissenschaftlich-ärtzlich Praxis*]" and that of "*philosophy*." Again and again, Heidegger will point out the need to be clear about this difference. He also brings up Sigmund Freud's psychoanalysis, whose "*assumptions*," i.e., presuppositions in the

---

1 Cf. the postscript to Martin Heidegger, *Early Writings* (*GA* 1) (Friedrich-Wilhelm von Herrmann, ed.) (Frankfurt am main[: Klostermann,] 1978), p. 437 f. [Translator's comment: Much has been written about the scholarly significance of this edition *letzer Hand*. The term means nothing more than based on the *original manuscripts*, whether they be in cursive script or Heidegger's brother Fritz's typescript or, probably very commonly, marked-up typescripts. In the years to come there will certainly be critical editions of books and essays Heidegger published during his lifetime and perhaps also of the numerous volumes of other material from the *Nachlaß*, including these seminar notes.]

D. The Zollikon Seminars

natural sciences, are often discussed. It is notable that in his explanations Heidegger does not just first return to *Being and Time* but refers to his current relevant thinking.

The second seminar, held on February 3, 1960, emphasizes the problem of "being with [*Mitsein*]" and he now focuses his thematic approach on *Being and Time*. Heidegger's term "sojourn [*Aufenthalt*]," often used in the "Zollikon seminars," first turns up. Heidegger recalls emphatically his elucidation of the "understanding of being [*Seinsverständnis*]," the foundation of the "analytics of existence [*Daseinsanalytik*]." He references Freud and discusses the concept of the "unconscious" as well as "slips [*Fehlleistungen*]." His interest in psychology extends, for example, to Viktor Emil von Gebsattel [1883-1976], the psychiatrist who had treated Heidegger in Badenweiler for three weeks in 1946. The last manuscript leaf of the seminar includes a list of the participants at the meeting of February 5, 1960.

The notes of his conversations with Medard Boss in Sicily in April and May 1963 refer to several topics [876] which are also discussed in the seminars. The concept of "sojourn [*Aufenthalt*]" is expanded to "world stay [*Weltaufenthalt*]." Heidegger repeatedly remarks on the "set-up [*Ge-Stell*]." The last notes [*Notate*] have to do with the question: "Is there an earth without man?" Boss left a record of the question and Heidegger's remarks about it in his own notations. While Boss often mentions his "India" experience in the latter (Boss had twice travelled to India before 1963), there is, however, no trace of India to be found in Heidegger's notations.[1]

The seminars of January 24 and 28, 1964, are the only ones based on one of Heidegger's own publications. In 1963, he had just brought out as an individual work his essay "Kant's Thesis about Being," which first appeared in 1962 in the *Festschrift* for Erik Wolf [1902-1977], *Existenz und Ordnung*. The seminars do not literally revolve around the essay, but rather take it as an occasion to revisit the relationship of Freud's psychoanalysis to natural science, and discuss it in its current and very general meaning—for example, in relation to the problem of "causality."

---

1 [Translator's comment: This is not quite right, since Heidegger refers to the 8th-9th-century Indian philosopher, Ari Shankaracharya, in his notes to the February 3, 1960 seminar just reviewed.]

D. The Zollikon Seminars

In the seminars of July 6 and 9, 1964, Heidegger builds on considerations of the January seminars by addressing an important problem of psychology and psychiatry. What role do causality and motivation play in human activity [*Praxis*], e.g., in the area of compulsions? In addition, the notes contain a self-criticism in which Heidegger admits that the "previous evening's seminar" "was unsuccessful [*mißglückt*]."

The seminars of November 2 and 5, 1964, take up the problem areas of the immediately preceding seminar. They are primarily about the self-understanding of contemporary and modern science, above all physics. Heidegger asks what sort of relation with nature is given expression in this self-understanding. Of particular importance should be a note that records a visit by Carl Friedrich von Weizsäcker [1912-2007] to his cabin in Todtnauberg, on September 19, 1964. The conversation was about "the unity of physics."

Quite obviously, on January 18 and 21, 1965, in his next encounters with Boss and his listeners, Heidegger made a shift [*Veränderung*]. For the first time, the problem of *time* is at the heart of his elucidations. It is identified as an important [877] phenomenon of psychiatry. There Heidegger refers in detail to his analysis of "boredom" from the winter semester of 1929/30 [lecture course] (*GA* 29/30) and interprets an essay on schizophrenia in which a "wall clock" is decisive. In general, in these notes Heidegger unfolds a broad field for the phenomenology of time in which the classical standpoint of the metaphysical philosophy of time, from Plato via Hegel to Husserl, is taken into account.

The eighth seminars, of March 10 and 12, 1965, are an unbroken continuation of the considerations of time. Attention is drawn more intensively to the scientific approach to the phenomenon of time in contrast to phenomenological investigations of an understanding of time, which are important for psychiatry. These studies also include the remarks on the "visualization" of Zürich Central Station. The rich notations on the subject that I have associated with these seminars also contain, for example, comments on the development of classical mechanics in Newton, the biology of time of Adolf Portmann [1897-1982], as well as Ernst Jünger's [1895-1998] *Sanduhrbuch* [*The Hourglass Book*] (1954). In general, it is amazing [*erstaunlich*] how many different texts and text citations Heidegger has drawn on.

D. The Zollikon Seminars

While the Zollikon seminars of January and March 1965 were devoted above all to time in relation to the experience of "existence [*Dasein*]," the Seminars of May 11 and 14, 1965, concern themselves for the most part with the body in its spatiality. For example, there Heidegger deals directly with discussions of "psychosomatics [*Psycho-Somatik*]" co-developed by Medard Boss. Thus, an essay from 1964 by Robert Marquard Hegglin [1907-1969], "Was erwartet der Internist von der Psychosomatik? [What Does the Internist Expect from Psychosomatics?]," is discussed. In addition, one finds here generous excerpts from Elisabeth Ströker's habilitation thesis from 1963, *Philosophischen Untersuchungen zum Raum* [*Philosophical Investigations on Time*], presented with critical remarks. Finally, it is striking that in his remarks on the body in its spatiality references to cybernetics appear for the first time (Heidegger cites essays by Gerhard Zerbe and is especially attentive to Nobert Wiener's book *The Human Use of Human Beings: Cybernetics and Society* from 1950, which appeared in German translation in 1952 with the title *Mensch und Mensch-Maschine.Kybernetik und Gesellshcaft*).

[878] The fourth seminars from 1965, held on July 6 and 8, contain the first notes on the question of method, especially the scientific method of measurement. In them, Heidegger finds an opportunity to make connections to cybernetics more frequently. Pertinent to notes on method in natural science and on cybernetics are a number of notations [*Notizen*] on technology, as well as commentary on Werner Linke [1907-1976] and Theodor Litt [1880-1962]. In counterpoint with these notes are others on the question of the "I-Thou relationship" or "others," described by Martin Buber [1878-1965] and Michael Theunissen, respectively. We find critical comments in relation to both positions.

In the fifth seminars of 1965, which took place on November 13 and 16, for the first time Heidegger deals in detail with the concept of "existential analysis [*Daseinsanalysis*]" as distinct from the "analytics of existence [*Daseinsanalytik*]." In this context, he occasionally refers to Ludwig Binswanger and Medard Boss.

In the seminars of March 1 and 3, 1966, Heidegger focuses on an important phenomenon of psychosomatics—stress. In this connection, he evaluates a "survey" from the *Zeitschrift für Psycho-somatische Medizin*, to which Heidegger often refers in his considerations from

D. The Zollikon Seminars

1965 on. In the context of the survey, he turns, for example, to the writings of Hermann [sic] Plügge [1906-1972].[1]

The notes from the last Zollikon seminars, held on March 18 and 21, 1969, deal with various things such as the difference between "consciousness and existence," "tautology," and "event [*Ereignis*]." Perhaps a pair of remarks about Herbert Marcuse [1898-1979] and his widely read treatise *Der Eindimensionale Mensch* [*One-Dimensional Man*] of 1967 can be understood as a reference to the *Zeitgeist*.

The minutes of Heidegger's remarks and conversations with participants as well as Boss's notes on his talks with Heidegger in Sicily can now be compared with Heidegger's notations [*Notizen*]. They appear interpolated here and there in Heidegger's marginal notes [*Randbemerkungen*]. Since in some places what is recorded in the minutes is almost identical with Heidegger's notes, it was impossible to avoid repetition.

*

[879] I have tried to reproduce as accurately as possible the character of the notes of the "Zollikon seminars." Drawings which appear to be part of the thematic as such have been included. References which Heidegger assembled in large numbers for the seminars were also taken into account. They are important because we learn from them what Heidegger took into consideration in preparation for the seminars: a lot of Freud, but also texts by Viktor Emil von Gebsattel, Medard Boss, Franz Büchner [1895-1991], Hermann [sic] Plügge, Robert Marquard Hegglin, Franz Fischer [1908-1999], Arthur Jores [1901-1982], Hans Binder, Werner Linke, Theodor Litt, Norbert Wiener, Gerhard Zerbe, Herbert Stachowiak [1921-2004], Carl Friedrich von Weizsäcker, Mircea Eliade [1907-1986], Ernst Jünger, Johann Wolfgang von Goethe [1749-1832], Henry Miller [1891-1980], Martin Buber, Herbert Marcuse, Elisabeth Ströker, Michael Theunissen, Joseph Conrad [1857-1924], etc. For some who are named I have given brief biographical references in footnotes or indicated text passages in their entirety that were cited by Heidegger. The notes were compared with the original publications

---

1 [Translator's comment: Trawny means Herbert Plügge.]

D. The Zollikon Seminars

and, if need be, corrected. Underlinings in quoted passages indicate Heidegger's own underlinings in addition to italics already found in the original.

Notes that pertain to certain publications (such as, for example, those on "boredom" in the lecture course *Die Grundbegriffe der Metaphysik. Welt—Endlichkeit—Einsamkeit* [*The Fundamental Concepts of Metaphysics. World—Finitude—Solitude*], GA 29/30, Friedrich-Wilhelm von Herrmann (ed.), Frankfurt am Main, 1983 and later editions) were provided with references to their respective places in volumes of the *Complete Edition*.

Heidegger's not infrequently sketchy notes were edited only very cautiously for orthography and syntax. Their character should be preserved. An illustration drawn by Heidegger (p. 27) was reproduced in the original; the other drawings were rendered schematically. Square brackets originated with the editor only when they indicate obvious omissions in sentences; all others are Heidegger's. Page numbers in square brackets indicate text passages in the GA that Heidegger cites in the manuscripts and for which he provides page numbers. The character □ is Heidegger's own abbreviation for "manuscript." The character [?] indicates a questionable reading. Illegible places are identified in the comments. Headings [880] in square brackets have originated with the editor as have the footnotes in square brackets. When commentary appears in footnotes without square brackets, it is Heidegger's.

*

Not Mr. Arnulf Heidegger, Esq., who was not yet the *Nachlaß* administrator for the *Complete Edition*, but his father, Dr. Hermann Heidegger, who on the advice of Professor Dr. em. Friedrich-Wilhelm von Herrmann assigned me the task of being editor of Volume 89 of the *Complete Edition* of Martin Heidegger. I thank Dr. Hermann Heidegger and Mr. Arnulf Heidegger for your unwavering trust in my editorial work.

I thank Professor Dr. em. Klaus Held for his support in the deciphering of some difficult-to-read passages and for his always friendly support in the coming into being of the volume.

D. The Zollikon Seminars

I thank Professor Dr. Guy van Kerckhoven (Katholieke Universiteit Leuven) for his indispensable help in deciphering Heidegger's handwritten notes.

I would like to thank Mrs. Jutta Heidegger and my doctoral candidate, Mrs. Kathrin Lagatie, for their intensive proofreading.

I thank Professor Dr. Alfred Bodenheimer, Dr. med. Klaus Rohr, and Professor Dr. med. Dr. phil. Ambros Uchtenhagen for permission to publish concise biographical information on still living as well as deceased participants in the seminars.

I would like to thank Mrs. Ruth Haener and Mrs. Barbara Stolba of the editorial archives of the *Neue Zürcher Zeitung* for providing a pdf file of its special issue published on the occasion of the 70th anniversary Martin Heidegger's birthday.

I thank Ms. Privat-Dozentin Dr. Anett Lütteken, head of the manuscript department of the Zürich Central Library, and Ms. Cornelia von Arx Schwan, the administrator of Medard Boss's *Nachlaß*, for information about his literary remains.

Wuppertal, September 12, 2017   Peter Trawny

b. Discrepancies between GA 89 and the Boss Edition of Zollikoner Seminare[1]

First, a few comments on the Boss edition are in order. Most readers will be familiar with the English translation and it is readily available in a paperback edition, the only book still in print (even on demand) bearing Boss's name.

The editors of the "American translation" acknowledge the participation of Joseph J. Kockelmans (mistakenly given as "W. Kockelmans") and William J. Richardson as early consultants in the project. Fr. Richardson's part was probably more extensive that suggested. In her conclusion to the translation's preface, written after Boss's death,

---

1   Appendix A contains a chart comparing the contents of the three volumes—*GA*, *ZS*, and *TR*. Appendix B details the table of contents for each of two German editions as well the section headings for the translation. They are provided as a convenient map and orientation for study of the two editions of the seminars, especially if the reader does not have ready access to the *Complete Edition* volume which retails at over $100.00 as a single volume, not including shipping.

D. The Zollikon Seminars

his widow, Marianne Boss-Linsmayer, notes: "It was not granted to Medard Boss to participate in the progress of this translation and to review the final text. Fortunately, Professor William J. Richardson (Boston College) undertook this task" (*TR* xii). Is it therefore reasonable to add his name to those of Franz Mayr and Richard Askay as ultimately responsible for the translation decisions and 239 footnotes of the edition?[1] Also acknowledged are Thomas Sheehan, Michael Zimmerman, and Calvin Schrag for their roles in reviewing parts of the translation. Finally, we read that Suzanne Mayr, MA, "edited and reworked the final draft of the English translation" (*ZS* vii). It is not clear what was entailed in such "editing" and "reworking" of what Mayr, Askay, Richardson and others had prepared.

Of interest is an acknowledgement of Heidegger's son, Hermann Heidegger, "for his support of our translation" (*TR* vii) since it would be the very same Hermann Heidegger who about fifteen years later was also thanked by Peter Trawny for his "unwavering trust" (*GA*, 880) in Trawny as editor of the *Complete Edition* volume. In his preface to the first German edition (dated "Spring 1987"), written when Boss was 84, he, too, acknowledges the support of Heidegger's son, who was then the literary administrator of Heidegger's *Complete Edition*. The *Zollikoner Seminare*, he writes, were scheduled for publication "at a much

---

[1] William J. Richardson was the most important early scholar to make Heidegger available to American students of Heidegger's thought. He was also a mostly Lacanian psychoanalyst. His article, "Heidegger among the Doctors," in John Sallis (ed.), *Reading Heidegger. Commemorations* (Bloomington: Indiana University Press, 1993), pp. 49-66, is still the best "review" of *ZS* in its clarity and understanding of the humanity of both protagonists in the Boss-Heidegger collaboration. In an interview in 2005, Fr. Richardson said: "[Heidegger] did work on clinical cases and had [some idea] of clinical experience. His knowledge came mainly from Medard Boss. The relationship between Boss and Heidegger became a friendship, rare in that age. Boss found Heidegger's existential analytics very attractive. He first got to know Heidegger's thought around 1940 and they began to take trips together after they got to know each other. Heidegger was near Saint Moritz and regularly traveled to Switzerland to teach there at Boss's request." "On Heidegger to Lacan. An Interview with William J. Richardson, SJ, PhD," in *Acheronta. Revista de Psicoanálisis y Cultura* **22**, December 2005: http://www.acheronta.org/reportajes/richardson-en.htm Professor Sheehan was unable to recall his contribution to the project (personal communication).

D. The Zollikon Seminars

later time" (-/XVI/xxi)[1] in Part IV ("Comments and Notes") of the *Complete Edition*, which had begun publication a little over ten years earlier. But this was an exceptional publication. Friedrich Wilhelm von Herrmann, Hermann Heidegger's "expert collaborator [*sachkundige Mitarbeiter*]" (-/XVI/xxi) and Heidegger's last academic assistant, Boss notes, "gave me, Dr. Heidegger, and the publisher, Mr. Michael Klostermann, the idea of publishing the *Zollikon Zeminars* ahead of schedule as part of the *Complete Works*" (-/XVI/xxi—Mayr and Askay choose "works").

Boss explained why this unprecedented exception was made: "It is highly improbable that the present editor will be alive in the next decade" (-/XVI/xxi). In the very next sentence, he wisely cautioned: "At the same time, it is difficult to imagine how someone could arrange and prepare for publication the shorthand seminar notes [*Stenogramme der Seminare*], the dialogues, and the letter excerpts" (-/VVI/xii). It is not clear that he was referring to the copious material we find in *GA*. Boss also expresses his indebtedness to Professor von Herrmann for "the preparation of the very detailed table of contents" (-/XVI/xxi). This was said to be Heidegger's wish *in lieu* of an index for all volumes of the *Complete Edition*. The preface concludes with Boss's thanks to Marianne Boss-Linsmayer for "her expert cooperation in organizing, and selecting from, Heidegger's papers" (-/XVI/xxi). It is not clear what material Mrs. Boss had access to and reviewed when she worked with "Heidegger's papers."[2]

Given that Professor von Herrmann also assisted Trawny, the presence of the September 8, 1959, seminar in *ZS* and the absence of one dated November 1959 which appears in *GA*, one must assume that between the late 1980s and the late 'teens of the present century,

---

1 From this point on, I will cite page numbers with three volumes in mind and in this order: the two German editions—*GA* 89 [= *GA*] and Boss's *Zollikoner Seminare* [= *ZS*]—and the English translation [= *TR*] of *ZS*, even when this tedious. When material is missing from a volume, including the translation, a "-" is given in its place. I abandon the convention, however, when it is obvious that a peculiarity of only one volume is being pointed out.

2 This preface is one of several places where Boss defends Heidegger against allegations of being a "typical Nazi [*Nazi-Mann*]" (-/VIII/xvi) that were made about him soon after World War II and continue to this day. A better translation might be "a Nazi guy" or "one of your typical Nazis."

D. The Zollikon Seminars

some archival material has gone missing and/or new manuscript material was located. During the late 1970s Heidegger's Nachlaß first began to be transferred to the German literary archives in Marbach, a process that is evidently still ongoing.

Regarding the *Gespräche* (1961-1972), Boss writes that given the great amount of time he and Heidegger had spent together during Heidegger's stays in Boss's home and while traveling, there was ample opportunity for dialogue [*Zwiegespräche*]. Boss writes: "It finally occurred to me to take down Heidegger's statements [*Aussagen*] in shorthand [*mitzustenographieren*] . . . . Understandably, I was able to record only a fraction of what was said during the discussions [*Diskussionen*]. This collection of shorthand notes [*Stenogramm-Sammlung*] forms part 2 of this book" (-/XIII-XIV/xix).

Boss also tells the reader about a correspondence of 256 letters and more than 50 postcards from Heidegger that he received between 1947 and 1971. Excerpts from these comprise the third part of ZS [*Briefe*] but only 110 of them are represented: 31 from before the seminars began, 69 from during the period 1959-1969, and 10 from during the last seven years of Heidegger's life (-/299-362/237-291).

Before continuing to compare the two editions, we turn to Boss's account of how the material published in the first part of his edition of *Zollikoner Seminare*, the minutes [*Protokolle*]), was gathered. In the Mayr/Askay translation:

> The seminar protocols recorded by students were unsuccessful [*mißerfolge*], so I took over the recording [*Protokollführung*]. Beginning with the next seminar[s], I recorded Heidegger's every word [*wortwörtlich jede* Äusserung *Heideggers*].[1] I dictated the

---

1 According to Trawny, the student who took notes at the first seminars at Boss's home was Erna Hoch, MD. Boss has the Zollikon seminars beginning with the week of July 6 and 9, 1964 (see 669-690/10-29/8-24). Since the meetings of January 24 and 28, 1964, were devoted to Heidegger's paper "Kant's Thesis about Being" that would mean Boss "took over" beginning with the November 1964 meetings. Trawny notes that his archive source (B74,1) contains material on the Kant paper seminar along with "minutes from July 6 and 9, 1964" (GA 873). Minutes are preserved in ZS only beginning with the January 1964 sessions. The Hoch notes identify Heidegger (H.) and a student (S.) and, in this case, it seems that indeed "Heidegger's every word" was recorded, much as a court stenographer might do. Beginning with the

D. The Zollikon Seminars

short protocol [*Stenogramm*] into a tape recorder immediately after the seminar.[1] Then my secretary transcribed it into typewritten form. Next the protocol drafts were immediately [*regelmäßig*] sent to Heidegger in Freiburg. He corrected them very carefully, made some minor additions here and there [*da und dort*], and occasionally added major additions in his German handwriting. He returned the corrected and supplemented protocols to me. Finally, these fully authorized protocols, corrected by Heidegger himself, were mimeographed in typewritten form [*Reinschrift*] so that every seminar participant had a record of them and had a chance to prepare for the next seminar (-/XII/xviii).[2]

We will return to Erna M. Hoch, MD, the "student" who was relieved of taking notes, in connection with Boss's "India book."

One additional comment found in the preface on Heidegger's presence during the seminars is relevant. Boss speaks of Heidegger's "unwavering patience and forbearance [*nie erlahmenden Geduld und Langmut*]" in the face of the evident incomprehension of most of the seminar participants. For Boss, in *being* so, Heidegger showed "the highest level of human fellowship [*der höchsten Form der Mitmenschlichkeit*]" exemplified by "selfless, loving *solicitude, which leaps ahead* of the other [human being], returning to him his own freedom" (-/XI/xvii). Lost in *TR* is what one would recognize immediately as a reference to the form of caring or looking after [*Fürsorge*] unique to

---

November 1964 minutes, however, we find summaries instead of the record of a dialogue.

1   It is curious that Boss did not audiotape the seminars even though the technology was available. Perhaps Heidegger objected.
2   Boss tells us: "Numerous proper names were not printed in this book whenever such anonymity did not detract from the content of the particular passage. Nevertheless, some proper names could not be eliminated without making the whole context incomprehensible. In making each of these decisions, I obtained Martin Heidegger's approval during his lifetime [*holte ich jedoch nochzu Lebzeiten Martin Heideggers dessen Einverständnis ein*]" (XV/xx). Keep in mind that, as Boss reports, "each year, beginning in 1959, I invited from fifty to seventy colleagues and psychiatry students to seminars at my home on the occasion of Heidegger's two-week visits" (/X/xvii). By contrast, in *GA* (60-61 and *passim*) Heidegger's notes reveal the names of some of the participants.

D. The Zollikon Seminars

the existential analyst. Following Heidegger's terminology in *Sein und Zeit* ¶ 26, Boss here speaks of Heidegger's *vorausspringende Fürsorge* or way-making looking after for other human beings, which we know Heidegger contrasted with interventional looking after [*einspringende Fürsorge*], which also happens to be characteristic of medical practice, training, and governing. Does this not make Heidegger an existential analyst in his own right? Did Heidegger's seminars have about them a quality that was similar in some respects to an existentially-informed [*daseinsgemäßig*] therapeutic situation?

Returning to a comparison of the two German editions, it is worth repeating that, as Trawny wrote in his editor's postscript to GA, Medard Boss's *Nachlaß* were not available for inspection at the time he was working on edition. That is still the case, which makes it difficult to give any definitive explanations of some important discrepancies between the two editions.

The first of them is a drawing reproduced in *ZS* (-/3/3) and a brief text identified by Boss as "Heidegger's notation [*Notiz*]" (-/3/337]) on the drawing. Trawny did not find either item in the Marbach *Nachlaß*. Boss dates the seminar in which Heidegger is said to have made use of the drawing as December 8, 1959. It is also not clear whether, as Boss said, a "verbatim protocol of the entire seminar does not exist" (-/3/337), or whether it is perhaps still among uncatalogued material not unavailable to Trawny.

Next, the first two GA Burghölzli seminars (7-16/-/-) (also referred to there as the "Zürich seminars") are not mentioned in *ZS*. The session is dated "November 1959." It may be that Boss and Trawny are referring to the same event and Boss had mistaken the date. If so, however, Boss "notation" (-/3-4/3-4) and the GA "notes" should have certain themes in common. But they are different. Friedrich-Wilhelm von Herrmann's heading in the table of contents of *ZS* (-/XIX/xxiii) reads: "Das menschliches Dasein als ein Bereich *des Vernehmen-könnens*." *TR* reads: "Human Da-sein as a domain of the capacity to receive-perceive [*Vernehmen*] the significance of the things that are given to it" (-/-/xxiii). This does not correspond in any way to what Trawny provides.

We have also seen Trawny's overview of first of the two GA Burghölzli seminars. They are in two parts (based on Marbach B 56,

D. The Zollikon Seminars

6)—A: Zürich Seminar. November 1959, and B: Aristotle's *de anima* (412a3 ff.), where Heidegger defines ψυχή. The second Burghölzli seminar, dated February 3, 1960, is found in *GA* (21-61/-/-), but there is no reference to such a meeting in *ZS*. On this, Trawny's *précis* should be considered in connection with his list of manuscript sources. The material comes from the same archive folder and what is contained in it should be related material, since we are given to believe that Heidegger carefully organized the entire body of manuscripts before his death. The first item in the relevant folder (notes for the upcoming session) is dated by Heidegger. The second is given a title by Trawny: "Notes of the Burghölzli Seminar." The first (21-27/-/-) includes fascinating observations on what a seminar is. Here Heidegger refers to the last sentence of a lecture he gave at the conclusion of a seminar on Hegel's *Science of Logic* 1956-1957, "The Onto-theological Constitution of Metaphysics": "A seminar, as the word implies, is a place and an opportunity to sow a seed here and there, a seed of reflection [*ein Samenkorn des Nachdenkens*] that may at some point bloom [*aufgehen*] in its own way and bear fruit" (21, n. 1/-/-).[1] Although Heidegger's image is drawn from the flora phylum, the root of the word was likely not lost on most doctors in the audience: *semen* (sperm).

The initial seminar, then, was about *seminars* and there was little of clinical interest to the psychiatrists and psychotherapists who made up the audience. Indeed, Heidegger speaks of the ongoing seminar hour as an *Art Luxus* (21/-/-)—a sort of luxury. In the course of these notes, he refers to a recent (1959) book by his colleague the physicist Werner Heisenberg [1901-1976], references Freud's metapsychology paper on "The Unconscious" (1915), and quotes Descartes' *Meditations* and Georg Christoph Lichtenberg [1742-1799], an author for whom he had a special fondness.

Several diagrams are included: one depicts being-with [*Mit-sein*]; another is a crude, handwritten drawing of someone taking a photograph, illustrating how he saw Freud's model of the psychical system,

---

[1] Heidegger cites a page in his book *Identität und Differenz*, now *GA* 11 (Frankfurt: Klostermann, 2006, p. 79), from which Trawny quotes the relevant sentence. The lecture was given on February 24, 1957, at his cabin in Todtnauberg, a truly intimate setting.

D. The Zollikon Seminars

which interposes something artificial between the human being and what is there [das Seiende] in the world. More important are the notes from the seminar (32-61/-/-) itself which include a list of participants.

Trawny has provided headings for most of what is found in these twenty pages of manuscript, the first of which is "on existential analysis [Daseinsanalyse]." Annotated as "transcribed shorthand," the English phrase "temporal emergent" is given in parentheses (31/-/-). Was there perhaps an English-speaking participant? Referenced during the session are Nicolai Hartmann, Viktor von Weizsäcker and Viktor von Gebsattel, whose personal connection with Heidegger has been noted. Named contributors to the seminar are "Dr. Condrau" and von Gebsattel himself. There is a remarkable section on sleep, dreaming and wakefulness, headed by the editor "Meditation," in which Heidegger mentions the 8th-century Indian Hindu scholar of Vedanta, Adi Shankaracharya [788-820].[1] Heidegger shows some familiarity with Freud, referring to the introductory lectures on psychoanalysis and Freud's autobiographical study.

Following the notes and concluding the material for the second Burghölzli seminar is a text, dated March 1960, identified by Trawny as "Subjectivity, Consciousness and There-being." This certainly represents a different session, yet it is included in the subsection dated February 3, 1960. A section Trawny heads as "seminar notation [Seminarnotiz]" brings the February 3, 1960, section to a conclusion. The theme is consciousness. Reference is made to Edmund Husserl's *Logical Investigations* (1900), in particular the fifth, "On Intentional Experiences and the 'Contents.'" Contributions by a number of the participants are noted: Hans Kind, Gion Condrau, Jacqueline Bodenheimer [1923-1987], Gustav Bally, [?] Heydt, Fritz Meerwein, Edwin Blickenstorfer, and [?] Helfenstein.

The editions are incongruent in two other places:

(1) Boss presents the first of his conversations with Heidegger as occurring one day after "the seminar on hallucinations." The conversation is dated November 29, 1961, which means the seminar occurred on November 28, 1961 (a Tuesday). This text does not appear in *GA*.

---

1 As we will see, the Indian philosopher and poet plays an important role in the background of the discussion of Boss's existential analysis.

D. The Zollikon Seminars

There is, however, a gap in Trawny's list of sources between the March 1960 seminar and the source materials for 1963 (Taormina).

(2) Next in order of presentation of its material, the *GA* edition places notes of "Conversations with Medard Boss in Sicily, April 23 to May 4, 1963," which are not included as part of the second part of *ZS* ("Conversations"). These notes and what Trawny publishes as the minutes of their first seminar were found together in one place (59,3) in the Marbach archive. Only four sections of the material have Trawny's heading "Notations on Conversation with Boss." Six of the 17 sections have Heidegger's headings.

Two items are missing from *GA* that appear in Boss's edition: (1) A conversation (-/195-196/151-152), which is found only in *ZS*, clearly belongs to an exchange in Zürich, not Taormina. It likely refers to the same seminar on hallucinations already mentioned. The brief dialogue is about the hallucination of a male patient, presented by one "Dr. F." The discussion may be compared with Heidegger's phenomenological exercise of visualization (*Vergegenwärtigung*) of the Zürich train station during the seminars held March 10 and 12, 1965 (741-764/73-96/56-75) and to some of the extensive notes in *GA* (261-272/-/-) prepared for those seminars. (2) Two conversations, from September 7, 1963 and September 8, 1963, are also missing from *GA* (-/228-231/182-185). The *GA* notes for this section (66-84/-/-) are, however, unique to the edition. The first is notable for Heidegger's brief remark about children (-/182/228). The *GA* "minutes" and corresponding *ZS* "conversations" (629/197-226/153-181) are nearly identical, including what is reported about the May 5, 1963, airborne exchange between Boss and Heidegger *en route* from Rome and Zürich (666/227/181).

The seminars dated January 24 and 28, 1964, are treated differently in the two editions (89-110/5-9/4-8). In *ZS*, they are presented as the minutes of the second seminar (the first to be held at Boss's home), while Trawny uses Heidegger's manuscript label "Phenomenological Seminar with Medard Boss, January 24 and 28, 1964, in Connection with my paper 'Kant's Thesis about Being.'" Heidegger's folder (74, 1), which also contains minutes of the July 6 and 9, 1964 seminars (6 sheets), refers to "the paper" (37 sheets). It would seem that in *ZS* Boss has published his own notes for the sessions or made use of manuscript material not available to Trawny. The *GA* notes are quite detailed,

D. The Zollikon Seminars

while what readers have from Boss is quite brief. In *ZS*, there is reference to two of the participants (one "Dr. R" and a "Professor H").

Only with the July 6 and 9, 1964 sessions do the two editions more or less align. Two manuscript sources for the July 9 session are used by Trawny. In all, the notes in this section (V) are quite limited (115-137/-/-). Here Trawny first presents a series of notes headed "Causality and Motivation. Foundations" and then two other brief sets of notes from a different folder. Another set of notes for the second session, on July 9, 1964, also taken from a different folder round out what is found in the section.[1] Boss presents the two sessions in dialogue form (as recorded by Erna Hoch), which Trawny presents as minutes II (669-690/10-29/8-24).

The two sets of minutes are nearly identical for the July 6 session (669-681/10-20/8-17) and for July 9 (681-690/20-29/17-24), with the exception that in *ZS* Boss is identified apart from other participants in the dialogue. This is not carried over in *TR*. Then there is the session, we will recall, that Trawny singles out as containing an admission on Heidegger's part that the previous session (July 6) had been "rather unsuccessful [*eher mißglückt*]." In the other version of July 9, Heidegger is supposed to have said: "Die vorige Seminarabend ist mißglückt" (*GA* 135). Boss's transcript had begun with the words: "Letztes Seminar ist eher mißglückt." *TR* reads: "The last seminar was rather a failure" (681/20/17).

---

1   As Trawny notes, this text was previously published in *GA* 73.2, *Zum Ereignis-Denken* [*On Eventuality Thinking*] (2013), pp. 1375-1378, also edited by Trawny, which references Boss's edition (/20-29/17-24). The text, which is a heavily edited version of Boss's minutes, is included in Part VI of *Zu Ereignis. Ontologische Differenz und Unterschied* [*On Eventuality. Ontological Difference and Distinction*], in section IX, *Der Holzweg—Ontologische Differenz* [*On the Trail—Ontological Difference*], where it is given it special place in the subsection *Der Holzweg der Seinsfrage. Zur ontologische Differenz (Transzendenz)* [*Tracking the Question about Being. On the Ontological Difference (Transcendence)*] headed "Die Unterscheidung (Aus den Zollikoner Seminaren) [The Differentiation (From the Zollikon Seminars)]." None of the comments of the seminar participants are included in either of the *GA* texts. In his editor's postscript to *GA* 73.2, Trawny refers to "*GA* 99," "the so-called four notebooks from 1947" which eventually morphed into the *GA* 94-96 *Überlegungen II-VI*—the much discussed "black notebooks."

D. The Zollikon Seminars

Given its preamble by Heidegger, the seminar deserves our special attention. The attempt to make up for it consists of some of the most cogent critique of modern and contemporary natural science, including quantum physics, Heidegger brings to the seminars. Early on in the session, Heidegger is quoted as saying: "Science is *the* new religion" (681/21/18).[1] Indeed. The minutes for these sessions are the last to be presented in dialogue form.

The *GA* note for the seminars that met on November 2 and 5, 1964, are again sparse. They are based on four items collected in the same folder and given headings by Heidegger. The most interesting of them is "Das Nächstliegende [The Nearby]."

The seminars of 18 and 21 January, 1965 (*GA* seminars VIII), focus on time. Heidegger's notes on the topics of these meetings and those for the next two series are especially relevant for the third part of the present contribution, which is the nature and future of therapy, in particular the transitional form known as Boss's "da-seinanalysis" on the way to dasein-therapy or simply *therapy*.

Heidegger's notes (179-229/-/-) are taken from a folder headed "The Question Concerning Time I." Trawny refers to the section on boredom ("Langeweile und Zeit [Boredom and Time]") (219-229/-/-) in *GA* 29-30, *Die Grundbegriffe der Metaphysik. Welt—Endlichkeit—Einsamkeit*, Heidegger's Freiburg lecture course from the winter semester of 1929-30. *GA* minutes IV and Boss's account (his *fifth* seminar report) are, once again, nearly the same (711-738/45-72/36-56), with the exception that Heidegger's annotations are for the first time included in the minutes sections of *GA*.

The March 10 and 12, 1965, seminar meeting notes (*GA* Seminar VIII) are extensive (235-377/-/-). The corresponding minutes (741-764/73-96/56-75) in the respective editions are the same. In the notes, partly preparatory material and partly a record of what went on during the meetings, we find four subsections headed "On Time" (Trawny's headings), the second of which is devoted in part to "Hegel on Time." These notes, which, broadly speaking, consider the notion of lived time (vs. clock time) will prove to be as important for the therapist as it was for the existential analyst [*Daseinsanalytiker*].

---

[1] The American translators emphasize 'is' rather than 'the', as Heidegger does.

D. The Zollikon Seminars

The extensive session notes for May 11 and 14, 1965, concern Heidegger's understanding of spatiality and the body (383-466/-/-). This is reflected in the minutes (*GA* VI) (767-789/97-120/75-92) of the meetings. The notes for July 6 and 8, 1965, which first take up the topic of method, are likewise extensive (471-557/-/-). As noted by Trawny, there is discussion of Buber's I-Thou relationship (e.g., 555/-/-). The American novelist Henry Miller [1891-1980] is mentioned in the notes (535/-/-) for seminar X.

The *GA* VII minutes (793-817/121-146/92-112) correspond verbatim in both editions. *GA* Seminar XI covers sessions dated November 13 and 16, 1965. The *GA* VIII minutes, however, are dated November 23 and 26, 1965 (821-847/147-173/112-132), corresponding to Boss's edition. Heidegger's very sparse notes (563-577/-/-) are headed "Daseins-Analytik. Daseinsanalyse [Existential Analytics. Existential Analysis]." The seminar was concerned with distinguishing Boss from Binswanger. Terminological ambiguities, which have plagued *Daseinsanalyse* from the start, are highlighted here. This is fitting, since what has followed for the most part remains entangled in a conflation of the two approaches.

For the period from the July 1964 sessions through the March 1966 sessions, Boss's "conversations" might be correlated with the minutes and compared.[1] The March 8, 1965 "conversation" is, in fact, a handwritten text, independent in theme, that does not follow the previous January's topics or anticipate upcoming seminar sessions.

For the most part the May 1965 *ZS* conversations overlap the seminar sessions and have some topics in common. The July 1965 conversations are three independent contributions, the last of which

1	Conversations	*ZS/TR*	Minutes	*GA/ZS/TR*
	8. März 1965, Zollikon	236-242/188-195	March 10/12 1965	741-764/73-96/56-75
	12. bis 17. Mai 1965, Zollikon	243-247/195-199	May 11/14 1965	767-789/97-120/75-92
	8. Juli 1965, Zollikon	248-252/199-201	July 6/8, 1965	793-817/121-146/92-112
	10. Juli 1965	251/202	July 6/8, 1965	"
	[Juli 1965]	251-252/202-203	July 6/8, 1965	"
	28. November 1965, Zollikon	253/203	November 23/26, 1965	821-847/147-173/112-132
	29. November 1965, Zollikon	254-257/204-206	November 23/26, 1965	"
	29. November 1965, Zollikon	258/206-207	November 23/26, 1965	"
	30. November 1965, Zollikon	259/207	November 23/26, 1965	"
	1965, Zollikon	260/207-208	[November 23/26, 1965]	"
	6. bis 9. März 1966, Zollikon	261-264/208-211	March 1/3, 1966	851-864/174-187/132-143

D. The Zollikon Seminars

reprises Heidegger's discussion of affects in his two-volume book *Nietzsche* (1960). The first part covers a variety of themes. The second refers to a report on recollection [*Gedächtnis*] from the Burghölzli meeting on July 10. It is not made clear that Heidegger was in attendance at the hospital then, but it seems likely.

The November 1965 sessions take up, in part, the scientific status of Boss's *Daseinsanalyse*. The related notes from the last three days of November following the seminars are especially interesting in covering Wolfgang Blankenburg's critique of Boss's form of psychotherapy. They include a few words on Boss's upcoming lectures in Argentina in 1966. Finally, the conversations following Heidegger's seminars in March 1966, which are on topics familiar to the seminars, seem to be selective of what must have been a productive visit by Heidegger.

The last two pairs of the Zollikon seminars occurred in 1966 and 1969. Both visits by Heidegger occurred in March. For March 1 and 3, 1966 (*GA* seminar XII), Heidegger's notes on stress and related topics are brief (583-616/-/-). So, too, are the minutes (*Protokoll* IX) (851-864/174-187/132-143). Three years later, the last seminars met. For March 18 and 21, 1969 (*GA* notes XIII) there are just a few scraps (621-631/-/-), the last of which mentions a book by Manfred Bleuler, Jürg Willi and Hans Rudi Bühler published in 1966. The minutes (867-870/188-191/144-147) are barely a few paragraphs for each session.

With that, the task of preparing for a critique of Boss's edition of the Zollikon seminars has been completed. Its purpose has been to encourage readers to study Heidegger's notes now available in the Trawny edition. Familiarity with them can only enrich our understanding of what went on in the upper rooms of the house on Bahnhofstraße in Zürich. It has also been a goal of this review of Boss's publications to attempt to clarify the terminological missteps that have tripped up readers of his work. As I have made clear, I believe a return to Boss is timely and if we can understand what he actually said, the direction he offered for psychotherapy could be heeded and followed, perhaps by a fresh group of therapists.

Part II
A New Beginning for Therapy

The point of the present contribution is to examine the origins of Medard Boss's existential analysis, which I take to be a turning point toward a new beginning for therapy. His personal life has received too little attention. I hope to have remedied that in a few of its details. I believe there is a much fuller story to be told, but that will remain incomplete while his personal papers are still unavailable for examination.

There is no evidence in ZS of a professional and personal crisis in Boss's life. In fact, however, there had been an extended period of self-examination and re-evaluation of his beginnings and well-established beliefs. The Boss I met for just an hour in June 1976 left me with the impression of a warm, centered, powerful, settled personality. By then he had completed a transformation, begun twenty years earlier, that only recently I have come to appreciate. Then in his early 70s, Boss had just published the third edition of his *Outline of Medicine and Psychology*. I had not read the book in the German original which I did only after studying the English translation in 1979, a few years after our meeting. I was aware of the "India book" but had not read it. I knew Boss chiefly as the author of *Psychoanalysis and Daseinsanalysis*, published in 1957, just following the personally powerful experiences he recounts in the "India book" published two years later.

In what follows I try to see Boss as a person and not only as the famous psychiatrist who had gained the trust of Martin Heidegger, with whom he experienced a complex relationship of mentor and student and perhaps even *mutual* existential analytic encounter. I will present what I have been able to put together about Boss's experiences in and of "the East" and what they mean for understanding the origins of his existential analysis. The basic text is, of course, *Indienfahrt eines Psychiaters*.[1] The surprising connections between what is recorded there and Heidegger's thought will not be overlooked. The trips documented in his "India book" were taken just before the beginning of Heidegger's seminars in Zollikon. With Boss's experiences in India in mind, a fresh perspective on the seminars is possible.

---

1   I will refer to *Indienfahrt einer Psychiaters* (Neske: Pfullingen, [1]1959; Freiburg: Herder, [2]1966; Bern: Huber, [3]1976 [with "Postscript"], [4]1987 [with a new introduction], [5]2006) [= *IP*] and *A Psychiatrist Discovers India* (London: Oswald Wolff and Calcutta: Rupa, 1965) [= *PI*].

A. Boss, Heidegger, and the East: *A Psychiatrist Discovers India*

Medard Boss visited India for five months in 1956 and returned again in 1958 for three more months. His first visit was supplemented by a five-week stay in Indonesia and a brief visit to Sri Lanka (then known as Ceylon). The first visit was in response to an invitation to teach in India, but it coincided with a deep spiritual and professional crisis in the life of Boss the man and the physician.

His account of the first visit takes up the bulk of the "India book" and provides context for what Boss has to say about the impact of his travels in the Near East on his work as a psychiatrist and *therapeut*. The first part of the book is a bit of travelogue but also serves as background for Boss's transition from being a visiting dignitary to a humble seeker who literally sat at the feet of several Indian mentors. Boss spent about eight weeks in all in ashrams overseen by two of these sages. He came to be guided and tutored in Hindu spiritual practices, including yoga and meditation. As a photograph in the last edition of the "India book" documents (4*IP*, Figure 11) his quarters in one place were not of the Hyatt sort.

Important sociopolitical changes were still in their early stages in India in the late 1950s following the country's independence from Britain a decade earlier. Boss was attentive to them, observant especially of the introduction of technology into the everyday lives of Indians of the professional caste. What stands out for the contemporary reader is that much of what Boss said about the effects of technology on the

A. Boss, Heidegger, and the East

people of India might have been written this year. I was surprised to learn from two young native Indian *emigré* colleagues that what Boss observed about his medical colleagues in the 1950s is still the case today. By day, they were fully "westernized," but when they returned home they were transformed into dedicated observers of an ancient spiritual heritage. This remains true, I learned, not only of health care providers but also engineers and individuals absorbed by IT.

The image of cell phones on the banks of the Ganges near where the dead are being cremated on funeral pyres is certainly more striking than what even he might have envisaged (see *4IP*, Figure 2). Then as now, cows were free to roam as they chose as they have for thousands of years (see *4IP*, Figures 1, 3). Today selfies are being taken and Youtubes are being produced about these animals. As Boss had learned from Heidegger, however, technology is not primarily about gadgets. It is about a relation to what is there.

Having traveled the thousand miles from northern to southern India, Boss also logged another few thousand miles on his visits to Sri Lanka and Indonesia, including stops in Java and on Bali. It is amusing to imagine the patrician Swiss psychiatrist dancing with a Balinese girl in the middle of the night to the accompaniment of gamelan music (*PI* 168-169). But it is moving to read about his encounter with a famous female sage, Anandamayi Ma [1896-1982] (whom he identifies as "Annandamoyee") (see *4IP*, Figure 8), and his profound deference to a scantily clothed yogi master with long, stringy hair, loincloth, and a mesmerizing gaze (see *4IP*, Figure 7). He also met an 11-year-old boy who had already been in a monastery for three years (*4IP*, Figure 5) and whose face showed a seriousness and maturity that is hard to imagine among American lads.

Speaking of these photographs, unfortunately, the thirteen wonderfully evocative color images included in the fourth edition (1987) of the "India book" and its important prefatory article "After Twelve Years" are not available to readers of the 1965 translation.[1] They humanize Boss in a way that even his most self-revelatory texts including his

---

1   I have scanned them for anyone interested in seeing a partial visual record of Boss's sojourn in India. No translations of the book have followed the appearance of the 4th edition.

A. Boss, Heidegger, and the East

self-portrait do not.[1] One must also look elsewhere than the English translation (which is in any case long out of print) for Boss's important 1976 postscript added for the third edition of his "India book."

Boss reports that he had already read a great deal of primary literature on Hindu philosophy and theology before his travels. This coincided with a time a number of years before his personal crisis and about the same time (1947) he first read Heidegger's *Sein und Zeit* (*PI* 12) in earnest. A curious if not fascinating coincidence.

He had learned some Hindustani, but all the conversations he records evidently took place in English, at times with the help of translators. As we will see, there are some inconsistencies about his reports of these *Gespräche*.

The accounts of a series of conversations with three of the eight sages he met and spent time with are extensive. He tells us that immediately following his meetings with them he would "note down" [*aufzeichnen*] (*IP* 160) what they had said. Even though these texts are presented as verbatim accounts of what he heard, given the amount of material quoted, much of what we read is surely Boss's paraphrase, "translation," and interpretation of what his interlocutors had said. In this regard, we might compare these conversations to the *Gespräche* or *Zwiesprache* with Heidegger between 1961 and 1972 which were also based on Boss's handwritten notes and published as Part Two of *ZS*.

The highlights of the "India book" are what Boss called three miracles [*Wundere*], experiences that led to essential insights that both responded to and, in part, effected elements of his self-transformation as a *therapeut*. The first was his realization of "an essential sameness in all people" (*PI* 180), no matter their cultural background or any accidents of genetic constitution. His "patient load" while practicing in Zürich was extensive, but once outside of the hospital setting it was fairly homogeneous in the German-speaking part of Switzerland. At the height of his career, nearly everyone, rich or poor, was Christian in the canton of Zürich, and about equally divided between Catholics and Swiss Reformed protestants. While in India, Boss lectured psychiatrists,

---

1   See his self-portrait, "Medard Boss," in Ludwig Pongratz (ed.), *Psychotherapie in Selbstdarstellungen* (Bern: Huber, 1973), pp. 71-106. My translation of this text is in *Existential Analysis* **30**(1), 2019, pp. 169-198.

A. Boss, Heidegger, and the East

supervised psychoanalysts in training, but saw patients who were Christian, Hindu, Muslim, and Buddhist.

Although Boss discusses hospital psychiatry in India and Europe, there is scarcely a word about psychotherapy until the final chapter of the book. In its first pages, however, he makes the observation that the "only person who should be allowed to be a psychotherapist is someone who is able to know the exact nature of man and to say how and what we are actually *in the world* [emphasis added]" (*IP* 13).[1] In the first sentence of the paragraph from which this statement is taken (the opening sentence of the book) he explicitly refers to the "modern psychiatrist" and his or her most recent "variety [*Spielart*] the psychotherapist" as being a medical doctor [*Artzt*]. As is still the case, to be a psychiatrist required, first of all, medical training—the MD—but one wonders how Boss felt about non-medical or lay psychotherapists. This issue is a part of Boss's biography that is of special interest today when most existential analysts are not medical doctors. We will return to this matter in considering the possible contradiction at the heart of existential analysis as both a form of psychoanalysis and a form of encounter between two human beings that, as Heidegger taught, had to transcend the medical model grounded in the natural sciences. Boss's colleagues in the hospitals of India were medical doctors, but the sages with whom he sat were not.[2]

---

1 A psychotherapist is "*der um die Verfassung des Menschen genau Bescheid weiß und zu sagen vermag, wie und wozu wir eigentlich auf der Welt sind*" (*IP* 13). Alas, the English translation we have says something very different: "The only person really entitled to be a psychotherapist is a *doctor* with precise knowledge of the essential constitution of man: a *doctor* who is in a position to say exactly how and why we are here on this earth [emphasis added]" (*PI* 9). This should give one pause about the translation as a whole. See the next note.

2 We are certainly off to a bad start with the available translation: "The modern psychiatrist, and the psychotherapist in particular, is a doctor . . . ." Indeed the book's lead sentence, in the Frey translation, is very misleading: "The modern psychiatrist, and the psychotherapist in particular, is a doctor with a special attitude to most of the mental and organic ailments which modern medicine still has to grapple with. He holds that these ailments are, basically, the results of false mental attitudes and ideal." Boss wrote: "*Der neuzeitliche Psychiater und vor allem dessen jüngste Spielart, der Psychotherapeut, ist ein Artzt, der glaubt, die Großzahl der seelischen und körperlichen Leiden, die der heutige Heilkunde noch ernsthaft zu schaffen machen, seien im Grunde immer nur die Folgen geistiger Fehleinstellungen und falscher Zielsetzungen.*" That is to say: "The

A. Boss, Heidegger, and the East

I would suggest that Boss's own education as a doctor had failed him and that is what drew him to the mentors he found in India even while there as a psychiatrist among psychiatrists. After medical school, experiences with Eugen Bleuler, Sigmund Freud, Carl Gustav Jung and many other major figures in the psychiatric and psychoanalytic establishment of his generation, Boss had realized that medicine does not inquire into man's nature but instead makes certain assumptions about human beings that are grounded in the natural sciences. But medicine is not concerned with existence or being-in-the-world. This Boss learned from his Indian mentors—and Martin Heidegger.[1]

A look at his early publications suggests that until Boss's reading of *Being and Time* and Indian philosophy, he was entirely at home with the medical model. Reading Heidegger *and* Indian philosophy around the same time set the stage for open admission of his doubts. "For me," he wrote, "it was all about the consolidation of the principles [*Grundlagen*] of our psychology and medicine, about a deepening and proper grounding of our anthropology [*Menschenkunde*], in order to gain a better, more measured insight into what man is about in his authentic essence and determination [*Bestimmung*]."[2]

And yet—the two-fold influence of Heidegger's fundamental ontology of existence and Hindu religious and philosophical ideas and practices were never enough for him to turn his back on protocols of medical practice. His thinking changed, however, and in the development of his version of *Daseinsanalyse* the crucial differences between a *therapeut* and a *psychotherapeut* as a "variety" of the species psychiatrist became clear to him. At the same time, as we have seen, for Boss *Daseinsanalyse* was always understood to be a form of Freud's

---

modern psychiatrist and in particular his most recent variety, the psychotherapist, is a physician who believes that the majority of mental and physical ailments that are still a source of trouble for medical practice today are always fundamentally only the result of spiritual maladjustments and mistaken objectives."

1 R. D. Laing (1927-1989), whom I would also term an existential analyst, also spent an extended period of time in India and returned a changed man.
2 Here again the available translation lets the reader down and even misleads him: "The main things at stake for me were a consideration of the intellectual foundations of our psychology and medicine; a deepening and proper grounding of our anthropology; and the gaining of better, more adequate insights into the real nature of man in relation to his essential being and destiny" (*PI* 88).

A. Boss, Heidegger, and the East

orthodox *Psychoanalyse*. And like Freud, Boss realized that therapy is a calling [*Beruf*] (not a profession), echoing Freud's talk of healing as one of the three "impossible callings."

Now things become interesting. Boss made statements such as the following, which one cannot imagine coming from a psychiatrist, psychoanalyst, or psychotherapist of his time—and even less of our own: "One now recognizes in every patient who comes in quest of help a portion and a manifestation of the divine, and one is happy that one is granted the honor of rendering aid. Now one need only let the patient sense the genuineness of this knowledge, until the latter thereby becomes aware once again of his own divine nature. Naturally, this entails the renunciation of any payment [*Honorar*], of any acquisition of personal possessions in general, as well as of any personal therapeutic ambition and pride" (*PI* 93). Two very different matters, both radical, are broached. I begin with the latter.

None of the mentors or sages with whom he sat in India charged a fee. None of them "made a living" at being with Boss or any other seeker. Did Heidegger charge a fee for his many hours of seminar leadership in Zürich? One of the crucial matters here, especially for Americans, will be the possible incompatibility of "running a psychotherapy business" (for example, as a limited liability corporation) and responding to a calling, whether it be that of a thinker (Heidegger), a spiritual mentor, or a *therapeut*. Elsewhere, I have argued for a complete declaration of independence of therapeutic practice from the medical establishment. This will be a requirement for therapeutic practice that is genuinely existentially-informed (*daseinsgemäßig*) and is, I believe, an unacknowledged implication of the practice of existential analysis. No money will be exchanged, no insurance paid. Psychiatry will, of course, remain a form of medical practice, in hospitals and in the offices of specialists, but the *therapeut* if he is to be a believer in the freedom of the other, must meet him or her in the context of encounter, not the exchange of a service for some sort of compensation—"naturally," as Boss says.

The reader may look at other sources for further clarification of the difficulties of making this transition, but its inevitability is assured. Interestingly enough, psychiatrists may be in the best position to be *therapeuts*. A psychiatrist could "make a living" as such a specialist

A. Boss, Heidegger, and the East

treating real diseases (epilepsy, Alzheimer's dementia, and the rest) much as surgeon or dermatologist does. This would be the source of his income, not sessions of existential analysis with another human being. Teaching or writing are other sources of income that would allow one to support himself but also be free to engage in the work of the *therapeut*. I have also dealt with questions of preparation for doing such work. They are similar to the question of how to prepare someone to be a thinker or musician or a sage or mentor. The answer is simple: direct transmission from one person to another, not a program or series of courses and final examinations. There is no international association of spiritual guides. There are no training programs, national examinations, or state licenses for mentorship. There are no guilds of thinkers. Like every genuine thinker, there is only one *therapeut* of a certain *Art und Weise*. There was one Freudian, one Jungian, and one Bossian. There are many professional philosophers out there—many of them—working in universities, but there are few thinkers. How does transmission in therapy work? We read on in the "India book" for the model of such transmission, which begins to look more like dialogue in thinking than medical practice.

Most important perhaps in the passage just cited is Boss's assertion that only given such an arrangement is there the possibility of the therapist's recognizing "in every patient who comes in quest of help a portion and a manifestation of the divine," which leads to "transmission of that recognition" to the other in order that "the latter thereby becomes aware once again of his own divine nature." But what has "manifestation of the divine" in a human being to do with the science of psychiatry, with its talk of neurons, neurotransmitters, psychotropic medications, ECT, and the rest? What has it to do with courses of treatment? Nothing whatsoever. And that's precisely the point. What, then, is the reward for the therapist? To make sense of the question and a possible response to it, we return to hear more of Boss's experience as recounted in the "India book."[1]

---

1 I have come to the conclusion that this, Boss's self-professed "favorite book" is his *magnum opus* and not the *Grundriß*, which was the fruit of the Zollikon seminars. One might argue that the *Grundriß* belongs among Heidegger's books, just as the Zollikon seminars are published with Heidegger, not Boss, as the author.

A. Boss, Heidegger, and the East

While in India Boss experienced some sort of enlightenment, perhaps in several phases. He explicitly links these with what happens in *classic* psychoanalysis, "the modern illumination method of the West." Like practices leading to enlightenment, "psychoanalysis is an experiential science in such a consummate sense that it can never be learned just by studying books. Really only the experiencing of it in one's own body and in one's own soul enables one sufficiently to see what psychoanalysis actually is and is capable of doing" (*PI* 165). This quality of *classic* psychoanalysis made it easier, I believe, for Boss not to abandon it entirely. His point is that both psychoanalysis and Eastern enlightenment are *of* and not *about* something. They are immediate, direct experiences. Reading about such experiences can never substitute for *having* them. I may read volumes on turning a cartwheel or playing the piano but only executing a flip or sitting at a keyboard and playing on the keys familiarizes me what each is. Early in their relationship, Heidegger had written to Boss (June 14, 1949): "Real [*wirklich*] thinking cannot be learned from books. It also cannot be taught [*lehren*] . . .."[1] The same can be said for real therapy and spiritual enlightenment.

Based on an *extended* experience, all three are empirical in the *literal* sense of the word. As the original Greek source root for empiricism, ἐμπειρία, makes clear, we are here in the world of perception and practice, not mere familiarity with terms or rote knowledge. Thinking and therapy are practices, like yoga. There is no goal, no knowledge to be gained, no information to be collected, filed away, or put to use. This is the sense in which Freud could speak of psychoanalysis as interminable—or, better, indeterminate. Similarly, one is a pianist only playing the instrument. For the American reader especially, we are here in the existentially-informed [*daseinsgemäßig*] world of William James's *radical* empiricism. It is difficult but necessary to keep such empiricism apart conceptually from the positivist empiricism of the natural sciences, the so-called experimental method, and such things as "data" and "findings."

I noted the absence of Boss's photographs in the English edition. Before providing that text and additional discussion of Boss's

---

1 *ZS* 301 / *ZO* 239.

A. Boss, Heidegger, and the East

self-transformation as it is related to the origins of existential analysis, it is worth noting two important *additions* that were included in the English edition only.

The first follows a long "transcript" of what Boss termed his second "Indian miracle" (*PI* 100-128).[1] This an important text for appreciating both where his mentors in India and Freiburg concurred but also what was perhaps the basic point on which Heidegger and Boss could not agree. Their inability to concur reveals Boss as not merely a blind follower of Heidegger, in the same way that he was not just an acolyte of Freud or Jung—or of the wise men he met:

> When the master had begun to explain the fundamental term of the highest Indian wisdom, the word *chit*,[2] I could hardly believe my ears. For I had heard him say things which often corresponded exactly, word for word, to phrases I had heard in the West from the lips of the philosopher Martin Heidegger. With redoubled caution, I then tried not to consider the meaning of the Indian wise man's statements in the light of my knowledge of Western, so-called "**existential**" philosophy [*Existenzphilosophie*]. Not at any price did I want to have them distorted by seeing them through this conceptual filter. By so proceeding, I was very soon able to recognize the underlying difference between Western *Daseinsanalysis* [*Daseinsanalyse*] and the Indian doctrine of *chit*. The former corresponds only to that Indian insight which the master had just characterized as a mere preliminary stage. At this stage—as I had just heard—man and man's luminating, opening-up nature is of necessity needed so that something like "**being** [*Sein*]" can take place, can arise and shine forth at all. In accordance with the highest Indian wisdom, however,

---

1   Not knowing whether Frey may have altered what Boss asked to be added, I have taken the liberty of cleaning up a few spots. I assume Boss wrote this and the other brief addition in English. I have bolded the problematic terms and suggested what Boss likely had with German in mind.
2   *Chit* had been defined by Boss's interlocutor as "the non-objectifiabe event of primordial, dawning brightening [*das ungegenständliche Ereignis des ursprünglichen, aufgehenden Erhellens*]" (*IP* 175). The English translation reads: "the non-objectifiable occurrence of the primordial, emergent, opening-up illumination" (*PI* 127).

A. Boss, Heidegger, and the East

chit, primordial illumination and opening-up, is said to be possible purely by itself alone. It is said not to have to make use of **human existence** [*menschliche Dasein*] as that realm which would grant the necessary luminated openness for the arising of that which has to be, for its shining forth and its coming forth into its **being** [*Sein*]. Nevertheless, despite this fundamental discrepancy, I remained greatly dumbfounded by the entirely unexpected, very far-reaching affinity between what very recent Western *Daseinsanalysis* and very ancient Indian wisdom recognized as the most profound 'ground' of **'being-ness** [*Seiendheit*]' as such, this "ground" being called "clearance," "openness"—*Lichtung* by *Daseinsanalysis*, and *chit* by the Indian philosophical tradition. Could it be that in quite another part of our earth, in the Black Forest of Germany, the same deepest insight into that which is trying to well forth? Could this be happening at the very time when it is about to be completely obscured and suffocated by the bustle of technology in India, where it dwelt for so many millennia in the knowledge of her wise men?

My Indian teacher, however, left me little time to explore these considerations any further. I heard him already go on to say:... (*PI* 128-129).

This interpolation was made in the midst of the Zollikon seminars, in 1965, when the English translation went to press. It is likely that Heidegger received a copy of *PI* so that Boss's homage to Heidegger was known to him. Boss would echo this addition ten years later, after Heidegger's death, in the 1976 preface to the 3rd German edition of the "India book" given below.

While not necessary for the occurrence of being, being "could only ever be represented as a becoming aware of something in the light of the essence of man [*im Lichte des Menschenwesens*]" (*IP* 176). But, for the Eastern sage, the brightening illuminates whether or not there is human attention to register it or anything brought to light by it, including any questioning human being. No *perception* is entailed that, as it were, makes use of such light to see something.

Boss's interlocutor refers to an "old simile [*Gleichnis*]" found in one of the *Upanishads* that "being [*Sein*] and thinking [*Denken*] go together

A. Boss, Heidegger, and the East

[*zusammengehören*] the way two bundles of reeds do, so that if one is moved away, the other also falls over" (*IP* 176, my translation). Here one cannot avoid recalling a fragment of Parmenides (Diels-Kranz 3): τὸ γὰρ αὐτὸ νοεῖν ἐστίν τε καὶ εἶναι: it is all the same with thinking and being.

In sum, in a "preliminary stage [*Vorstufe*]" known to Indian philosophy, existence is not necessary for the brightening spoken of. For Heidegger, however, there is no such preliminary stage. Instead, existence is necessary for be[-ing] [*Sein*] since man is the there [*da*] of be[-ing]—better: man is there for be[-ing]. Be[-ing] is thus beholden to There-being (*Da-sein*). A closer, more careful elucidation of the issue and this section of the "India book" (*IP* 174-176, *PI* 126-128) is required, since it is about a "place" where Boss and Heidegger could not quite meet, where Indian wisdom as Boss understood it and Heideggerian thought could not meet.

The second addition, a single paragraph, follows soon after in the same chapter of the English translation:

> *Brahman* never means anything else but the occurrence of the fundamental opening up of an illuminated, free realm which, in its turn, is the indispensable prerequisite for the possibility of **being-ness** [*Seiendheit*] as such, i.e. of anything shining forth, coming forth into its existence (*PI* 139).

Once again, we do not have a German original, since presumably Boss wrote the introduction in English. But it may have been "corrected" by Frey. Again, the context of the interpolation requires an elucidation that must wait for another time.

Apart from paying tribute to Heidegger and to the similarities between Hindu philosophy and Heidegger's thought, the additions are also important for the ongoing discussion between Boss and Heidegger on the relation between *Sein* and *Da-sein*. Here is the 1976 "Postscript" to the 3rd edition:[1]

> The present book, *A Psychiatrist's Sojourn in India*, was first published in 1959 by Neske (Pfullingen). In 1966 it was published

---

1 See Appendix V for the German text.

A. Boss, Heidegger, and the East

a second time in paperback, albeit in an abridged version, by Herder.[1] If now the author and even more the publisher agree to publish the book again in a third edition, two full decades after it was written and once again in its unabridged and unaltered original form, they must be convinced of two things: first, they have to be sure no substantive misconceptions contained in the first edition have come to light which must be corrected; second, they must be of the opinion that even today the book has not lost any of its relevance.

That both are the case may be considered proven by the following facts:

The author did not go to India again after 1958, yet he has remained in continual contact with his teachers and friends, especially the *Mahamahopadhyaya* [esteemed scholar] who is extensively quoted above and whom until his death a few years ago I could truly call my "guru." Much that confirms the correctness of what is in the text of this book the author learned along the way from the Swiss psychiatrist Dr. Erna Hoch, who at the author's instigation took over the management of a psychiatric clinic in northern India eighteen years ago [1958] and has worked in India since then without interruption. She is now professor of psychiatry at the University of Kashmir at Shrinagar and director of the university hospital there. Most important, she followed in the footsteps of the author in studying Indian philosophy and Hindu meditation and kept him constantly informed about her experiences in this regard, both by letter and during her occasional visits to Switzerland.

Furthermore, without interruption the author himself has carried out on a daily basis the meditative exercises imparted to him by his Indian teachers in accordance with the instructions received at that time. After experiences of this kind as well, he

---

1 The English translation was unabridged. I prefer to translate the title as *A Psychiatrist's Sojourn in India*. Interest in Boss's travels in India has drawn some recent interest. See Miraj U. Desai, "Travel as Qualitative Method: Travel in Psychology's History and Medard Boss' Sojourn to India," in *Journal of Humanistic Psychology* 54(4), 2014, pp. 494-507.

A. Boss, Heidegger, and the East

does not feel any inclination to make any changes or additions to the original text of the book.

Finally, last fall [1975] it was granted to the author to be invited to Japan for a considerable amount of time because many of the medical, philosophical, and theological faculties of various universities in Japan were highly interested in his "existential-analytic school." In that way the author came into close contact with the most highly regarded masters of Zen Buddhism. He even had the good fortune to take part extensively in meditative Zazen with a group of Zen Buddhist monks. It is precisely a comparison of his Indian experiences with Zen Buddhist practices and teachings and what has become outstanding about them that has made it possible for the author to confirm just how factually the Indian realities mentioned in this book are described.

The author considers only one single supplement to be appropriate and fruitful at this point and at the present time. In the previous editions of *A Psychiatrist's Sojourn in India*, the author said not a word about what was for him really the most surprising and deeply shocking experience that awaited him in India. His greatest surprise was that he heard from the mouth of his Indian interlocutors a great number of propositions which, word for word, seemed to have been taken from the existential-analytical work *Being and Time* by Martin Heidegger. The author knew very well, however, that Heidegger had not heard anything of the Indian insights, nor had the Indian sages heard anything at all about Heidegger. The author omitted any indication of this so far because he was afraid that by including this experience he would in an all too disruptive way break up the course of his depiction of the Indian realities and ways of thinking, which was his only concern.

The occasion for making good this omission today is a crucial question which a critic has since made public. Even given the author's assertion in the foreword to *A Psychiatrist's Sojourn in India* about having read all of the available literature including books by Indian scholars on ancient Indian insights into the basic constitution of man, into the nature of his world, and into the nature of the relationship between the two before his visit

A. Boss, Heidegger, and the East

to India, the critic could not shake the suspicion that the reading was consistently falsified by forcibly being pressed into the service of Western Platonist and neo-Kantian paradigms of presentation. And (so the critical question continued) before listening to the Indian sages, did the author of the *Indian Sojourn* not probably doff the spectacles of Western metaphysical Platonism and neo-Kantianism only to put on those of the equally Western fundamental ontology of Martin Heidegger?

What astonished the author most about this question was not so much that it was made at all, but rather the fact that it was made public only once as far as he knew. That there was indeed a great danger that the author could, in an existential-analytic sense, *mis*hear was all too conscious to him from the start. Heidegger's new discoveries had only impressed him deeply shortly before. Precisely in full knowledge of this danger, the author had been able to arm himself against it accordingly. The best proof of his impartiality in this regard may be that at the same time the author also became aware of the fundamental difference between Hindu and existential-analytical human studies. The deepest insight of the Westerner Heidegger into that which is is that in his basic constitution man consists in a globally unbridled ability to attend to what is encountering him. As questioning openness of this kind, man is claimed as that place of appearance without which nothing could be given. All, that is, which is and has to be needs such a sacred space in order to come to pass somewhere, to "dawn" in the fullness of its meaning, to be able to make its appearance and thereby come into its being.

On the other hand, the author heard from the Indian *Mahamahopadyaya* (and not only from him) about the quite different kind of experience mentioned in this book. According to him, there is clearly only "Brahman," the "great dawning", "clearing", "lightedness", "awareness" even *without* the essence of man.

After his return from India, when the author reported this formidable contradiction between the Indian sages and the Westerner Martin Heidegger, after a long, thoughtful silence Heidegger replied that what had just now been conveyed by the

A. Boss, Heidegger, and the East

author was for him simply not immediately experienceable and therefore could not count as the truth for him. Heidegger expressed this with just as much certainty as the Indian sages had previously shown the author of their knowledge of non-human-dependent Brahman as the most immediate and most certain meditative experience.

On the other hand, if the insights of Indian sages are unbridgeably far from those of Heidegger's fundamental ontology, what the author heard in India about a "lightedness," "Brahman" which is there without what is there, even independent of man, indeed independent of a god, of gods, or a deity, is in all the greater closeness to the original Hindu experience which, on its way to the East, changed into the Zen Buddhism of southern Japan.

Before reviewing this text further, it is worth pausing to say a bit about Erna M. Hoch, who is mentioned in it and also participated in the Zollikon seminars.

Hoch is not mentioned by name in ZS, but is identified in GA, where Trawny devotes a very brief footnote to her.[1] In fact, she played a much more significant role in the Heidegger-Boss collaboration at this time than Boss tells us. Erna Hoch was an important mediator between Boss and various Indian scholars in India where Boss had been a visiting professor. We learn from Hoch that she was Boss's "messenger between East and West" who had been sent by Boss to speak with Kanti Chandra Pandey (1898-1974) and other Indian scholars on Heidegger's behalf.[2] In her book, she recounts conversations in 1960 with Pandey, who was Professor of Sanskrit at Lucknow University, where Medard Boss had taught. She reports, however, that nothing was gained by probing Professor Pandey about possible equivalences

---

[1] "Erna Hoch (1919-2003), born in Basel. After a stint in England during World War II in the Women's Auxiliary Service, she studied medicine in Basel and specialized in psychiatry. Beginning in 1956, she worked in India, then between 1969 and 1980 in Kashmir. She returned to Europe in 1988" (*GA* 669).

[2] Erna M. Hoch, *Sources and Resources. A Western Psychiatrist's Search for Meaning in the Ancient Indian Scriptures* (Zürich: Rüegger, 1991). In her book, published soon after Boss's death, Hoch provides much to reflect on regarding what she takes to be four similarities and four differences between Western existential analysis and ancient Indian philosophy.

A. Boss, Heidegger, and the East

between certain of Heidegger's notions such as be[-ing] [*Sein*] and 'what is there' [*Seiendes*][1] and Sanskrit terms used in ancient books of Indian wisdom. Pandey was noncommittal, even evasive much of the time. She had also inquired about any possible terms equivalent to Heidegger's *Lichtung*[2] in connection with the special status of the human being as existence in relation with be[-ing]. Hoch, who knew both psychiatry and Indian philosophy, was disappointed by her interlocutors, but she nonetheless concludes that Heidegger's "teachings had decisive consequences for psychiatry and psychotherapy" (p. 291), but that these were quite independent of the sort of wisdom a guru could provide someone on the path to transcendence informed by Indian philosophy.[3]

As a result of what Hoch told him, Boss's hope was evidently disappointed that parallels could be established between ancient Indian wisdom and Heidegger's insights. Was Heidegger also let down by this news from Boss? In any case, Boss wrote: "Could it be that in quite another part of our earth, in the Black Forest of Germany, the same deepest insight into that-which-is is trying to well forth? Could this be happening at the very when it is about to be completely obscured and suffocated by the bustle of technology in India, where it dwelt for so many millennia in the knowledge of her wise men?"[4] Here Boss is

---

1 As noted earlier, what is clear enough in German about the relation between *Sein* and *das Seiende* does not carry over into English. Briefly, the substantive *Sein* is based on the infinitive *sein*, which is an abbreviated form of *seien*, the German verb suffix '-en' having been absorbed. I write my translation of the substantive be[-ing] and pronounce it /bi/. The bracketed suffix is a reminder of that the word is a participle and, more important, that '(to) be' should be understood as a *transitive* verb. *Seiende* spells out the German participial form of *sein* and substantivizes it.
2 The American translation gives *Lichtung* for 'clearing' instead of what we find in ZS: *Gelichtete* [lighted] (/XVI/xx).
3 Hoch refers to p. 176 of Boss's book, but these sentences were added by Boss for the 1965 English translation (p. 129).
4 India is discussed in Boss's "conversations," which are presented as the first *minutes* of the GA edition. As Trawny points out in his postscript, there is no mention of India in Heidegger's notations, which Trawny finds surprising since there is so much about his Indian experience in Boss's minutes and Heidegger knew Boss's book. There may be places in Boss's *Nachlaß* where Heidegger comments on Boss's experiences in the East. I wonder whether Trawny may not be familiar with the passage Boss added only for the English translation in 1965

A. Boss, Heidegger, and the East

defending himself against the charge that his existential-analytical "turn" was simply the result of having become intoxicated with Heidegger's philosophy. He dismisses the idea of a critic that he might have misinterpreted ("mis-heard") either Heidegger or Hindu philosophy or both. That said, he turns to the point of contention that had occupied Heidegger and Boss on the relation between *Sein* and *Da*-sein. Heidegger's reported comment after Boss's 1956 stay in India is decisive. What the Indian sages had said was, in Heidegger's words "simply not immediately experienceable" for him and therefore "could not count as true" for him.

The certainty of both mentors, however, was equally convincing. Perhaps the most telling of Boss's comments is that the influence of Heidegger's ideas on him had come *after* the time of his reading of Hindu philosophy, in fact, "shortly before" he wrote the "India book" in 1958-1959. This is reported in the context of Boss's declaration that he "knew very well that Heidegger had not heard anything of Indian insights nor had the Indian sages heard anything at all about Heidegger." This is probably not accurate about Heidegger. There is much to suggest that Heidegger had some familiarity with "Eastern philosophy" but, as in the aborted project of translating parts of *Tao te Ching* begun with Paul Shih-yi Hsiao in early 1946, he hesitated to pursue studies in areas where he had no understanding of the original language.[1] I do not think that Heidegger read Sanskrit, which means that all of his experience of Hindu philosophy was second-hand. By contrast, given the wide-ranging knowledge of Western philosophy shown by at least one of the sages Boss spent time with, Heidegger's thought may well have been known to him.

About as interesting as Boss's observations are about the similarities between what he heard from his mentors in India and what he had read in *Sein und Zeit* and heard from Heidegger during their time together is the reference to Zen Buddhism at the end of the postscript, since the

---

    in which Boss expresses what he sees as a remarkable similarity between what he had heard from Heidegger and what he had heard from Govind Kaul, his guru from Kashmir.

1 Paul Shih-yi Hsiao, "Heidegger and Our Translation of the *Tao Te Ching*," in Graham Parkes (ed.), *Heidegger and Asian Thought* (Honolulu: University of Hawaii Press, 1987), pp. 93-101.

A. Boss, Heidegger, and the East

8th-9th-century scholar of Vedanta, Adi Shankaracharya [788-820], is credited with having achieved the synthesis of Hinduism and Mahayana Buddhism that evolved into Zen. He is mentioned by name in Heidegger's notes for his seminar of February 3, 1960 (37/-/-) at the Burghölzli.[1]

We now come to what is perhaps the most revealing text about Boss's experience and what it contributed to the development of his existential analysis.

While gathering material for this study and a complete bibliography of Boss's writings, I came across the published transcription of a letter he wrote on November 23, 1970. Dated after the last of the Zollikon seminars, it belongs among personal documents relevant to the origin of existential analysis. It was written at a time when Heidegger and Boss were less in contact, for the most part because of Heidegger's declining health. Most important, the letter is further documentation of the spiritual crisis around 1953 that perhaps unconsciously encouraged Boss to accept invitations to visit India. Boss would visit Japan in 1975 where earlier experiences in India were revivified.

Boss's letter is to the editor of a book of poems by Govind [or Govand] Kaul, *Govind Amrit* (1975). Somewhat "cleaned up," it reads:[2]

---

[1] Just how much of Heidegger is "Eastern" has been a fascinating question for a number of scholars: Graham Parkes (ed.), *Heidegger and Asian Thought* (Honolulu: University of Hawaii Press, 1987); Reinhard May [1989], *Heidegger's Hidden Sources. East Asian Influences on His Work* (New York: Routledge, 1996); Hartmut Buchner[1989], *Japan und Heidegger. Gedenkschrift der Stadt Meßkirch zum hundertsten Geburtstag Martin Heideggers* (Sigmaringen: Thorbecke, 1989); Lin Ma, *Heidegger on East-West Dialogue* (New York: Routledge, 2008). See also Graham Parkes, "Heidegger and Japanese Thought: How Much Did He Know and When Did He Know It?," in Charles Macann (ed.), *Martin Heidegger. Critical Assessments*. Volume 4: *Reverberations* (London: Routledge, 192), pp. 377-406. There Parkes writes: "Heidegger appears to have had relatively little interest in Indian philosophy" (p. 400, n. 1). I think this may have been a premature conclusion, especially given Heidegger's interactions with Boss.

[2] "Foreword" to Govind Kaul, *Govind Amrit* [*Immortal Govind*] (Bombay: Prithwinath Niranjannath Pandit, 1975), pp. 1-2. Boss's "Foreword" is followed by a tribute to him, "Salutations to a Godly Man," by J.M. Kayande, to whom the letter was addressed. Kayande paraphrases Boss at one point. I think we should be cautious in accepting what Kayande says he observed and heard. Here is the text scanned from *Govind Amrit* for archive.org found at https://archive.org/details/GovindAmritKashmiriSwamiGovindKoul/page/n5. The reader may compare this with my "cleaned up" version.

A. Boss, Heidegger, and the East

At the age of about fifty [1953] I had reached the stage of a well-established and not unsuccessful psychiatrist and academic teacher.

Forward [sic]

At the age of about fifty I had reached the stage of a well established and not unsuccessful psychiatrist and academic teacher. Peoples [sic] thought of me as a lucky man. Inside, however, the despair had grown to an almost unsupportable degree. Many of the best authorities in my field had been my teachers. Still I lacked any real understanding about the essence and the meaning of human existence. Most of the patients who came to ask for my therapeutic aid complained in a more or less veiled and hidden form of exactly the same failing in knowing about the goal of their lives. Finally, I had to realize that the natural scientific approach to man enabled the modern scientist only to manipulate [with] the human body in an extremely skillful way. Manipulation as such though, is by far no proof at all for an adequate understanding of the manipulated matter.

This state of affairs forced me to seek help outside the western world. I went to India. I had been told the Indian saints and philosophers had searched [F]or the truth about man and his world during an unbroken chain of thousands of years.

I met a great many very learned and saintly Indian men and women. To all of them I shall remain deeply indepted [sic] for their help. The turning point of my life, however, only occurred when I was brought before **Swami Gobind Kaul** who had come down from Kashmire just at that time to Goregaon, Bombay. There was no possibility for him and me to talk to each other directly. All my knowledge of several lenguages [sic], including my preliminary studies in Hindi were of no avail. Swamij only speak [sic] Kashmiri. Nevertheless, from the very start of our encounter an immediate non-verbal, rather a preverbal understanding between **Him** and me had sprung up. in **His** presence the many torturing questions about man's existence and about Beingness as such were instantly stilled. A closeness to Godhead at once had opened up. Later on **Swamiji** showed me through the Goregaon frinds [sic] as interpreters the practice of meditation. Ever since I follow his advices [sic] without any break where ever I have to stay in this world. I never could have fulfilled my rather heavy tasks as a psychotherapeutic doctor and as an academic teacher without this fountainhead of mental strengths which I was so lucky to find in India.

I am happy to learn than **Mr. Prithvi Nath Pandit** of Goregaon is going to publish some two hundred poems by **Swamiu Gobind Kaul** of Kashmire. I am sure that this book will bring all those who have eyes to see and ears to hear closer to the only realm which really matters.

Medard Boss, M.D.
Professor of psychotherapy
Medical School, University of Zürich, Switzerland. 23rd Nov., 1970

A. Boss, Heidegger, and the East

People thought of me as a lucky man. Inside, however, the despair had grown to an almost unsupportable degree. Many of the best authorities in my field had been my teachers. Still I lacked any real understanding about the essence and the meaning of human existence. Most of the patients who came to ask for my therapeutic aid complained in a more or less veiled and hidden form of exactly the same failing in knowing about the goal of their lives. Finally, I had to realize that the natural scientific approach to man enabled the modern scientist only to manipulate the human body in an extremely skillful way. Manipulation as such though is by far no proof at all for an adequate understanding of the manipulated matter.

This state of affairs forced me to seek help outside the western world. I went to India. I had been told the Indian saints and philosophers had searched for the truth about man and his world during an unbroken chain of thousands of years.

I met a great many very learned and saintly Indian men and women. To all of them I shall remain deeply indebted for their help. The turning point of my life, however, only occurred when I was brought before Swami Gobind Kaul who had come down from Kashmir just at that time to Goregaon, Bombay.

There was no possibility for him and me to talk to each other directly. All my knowledge of several languages, including my preliminary studies in Hindi were of no avail. Swamij only speaks Kashmiri. Nevertheless, from the very start of our encounter an immediate non-verbal, rather a preverbal understanding between him and me had sprung up. In his presence the many torturing questions about man's existence and about beingness as such were instantly stilled. A closeness to godhead at once had opened up. Later on Swamiji showed me through Goregaon friends as interpreters the practice of meditation. Ever since I have followed his advice without any break wherever I stay in this world. I never could have fulfilled my rather heavy tasks as a psychotherapeutic doctor and as an academic teacher without this fountainhead of mental strength which I was so lucky to find in India.

I am happy to learn that Mr. Prithvi Nath Pandit of Goregaon is going to publish some two hundred poems by Swamij Govind Kaul of Kashmir. I am sure that this book will bring all those who have

A. Boss, Heidegger, and the East

eyes to see and ears to hear closer to the only realm which really matters.

Medard Boss, MD
Professor of Psychotherapy, Medical School
University of Zürich, Switzerland
November 23, 1970

The reference to Kaul is important because at one point in the India book Boss seems to attribute to the sage from Kashmir with whom he says he had many talks the statement that "the incessant practice of a being's state of mind worthy of the truth [*das unablässige Üben einer wahrheitswürdigen Wesensverfassung*] is much more important than all talk [*Reden*]" (*IP* 223, author's translation). Here we are, I believe, at a formulation that is decisive for understanding what Boss drew from his experience in India and translated into his understanding of therapeutic encounter in his existential analysis.

Like his encounter with Kaul, for Boss what was essential to therapeutic encounter with another is "an immediate non-verbal, [or] rather a preverbal understanding . . . in his presence." This was evidently Boss's English text. I want to take liberties with the passage in one place and that is with the word 'presence'. As I have suggested in other places, the point of therapy is nothing other than the recovery of a person's *present* [*Gegenwart*], the immediate now that flows out of his existence, the present that makes time.[1] The German word *Gegenwart* can be rendered with both 'present' (as compared with the past and future) and 'presence'. In his recollection of the meeting with Kaul, Boss writes about Kaul's "presence," which for contemporary readers has about it something mystical, magical, even surreal. We associate with it such ideas as charisma, even something otherworldly. I do not know whether Boss had *Gegenwart* in mind when he wrote 'presence', but I cannot avoid concluding that he meant something more than some sort of charismatic "vibe" or "feel," but rather an experience of Kaul's *present*, his time-making *now*. This experience may be followed

---

1 Miles Groth, *After Psychotherapy* (New York: ENI Press, 2016; 2nd ed., Adelaide: YCH Publications, 2017).

A. Boss, Heidegger, and the East

by attempts at verbal articulation or it may remain at a "non-verbal, rather a preverbal" level. Much is communicated in silence.

As expressed in his letter, an "understanding" "springs up" in such encounter. This, by the way, is the sense of *springen* that, I believe, infuses the meaning of the way-making [*vorausspringend*] looking after [*Fürsorge*] that wells up in therapeutic encounter. The *therapeut* can offer only his own present to the greatest extent possible, bearing in mind that the goal for the other of therapy is nothing other than recovering his or her own present. The coincidence of two existences, of two such "presents," is what Heidegger understands by the term co-existence [*Mit-dasein*] in his fundamental ontology of existence. It is usually superseded and obscured by an incursion of talk. In traditional psychotherapy, this is usually in the service of reverting to past experiences or making plans for engineering a future. Therapeutic encounter is an unusual situation indeed, where human co-existence can be glimpsed. With this view of therapeutic encounter in mind, I believe, we can see what may lie ahead for a "real" existential analysis.

I add here as context Kayande's "Salutations to a Godly Man," which follows Boss's "Foreword." The veracity of the account remains to be attested, perhaps by documents in Boss's *Nachlaß*. If it is accurate, there is in it a picture of Boss that adds to our understanding of the depth of his existence.

Again somewhat doctored up, it runs as follows:

> Within that month one Dr. M. Boss, [an] internationally known psychiatrist of Switzerland happened to come to Bombay. Besides his professional engagements he had a secret mission of meeting realized souls in India. Someone in Benaras had advised him to find such a person in Kashmir. In the meanwhile he was introduced to me to discuss Advaita [Vedanta] and Yoga. He felt happy in my company and changed over from [the] Taj Mahal Hotel to Goregaon, [a] suburb of Bombay. Here at my place the illumined soul from Kashmir was sitting in my house. Dr. M. Boss with all his spiritual humility paid respects to him and within a few seconds something awakened in Dr. Boss's heart and he prostrated himself at the Swamiji's feet. The Swami embraced him and blessed him. No words were used, no efforts to convince each other. Dr. Boss

A. Boss, Heidegger, and the East

found the solace of his heart and God had used me as the mediator of the light. Dr. Boss writes from Switzerland [that] the Swamiji is "always with me in my mind as well and that I am doing Raj Yoga without any break as he has taught me, no matter whether I am, in America, in England, or on the continent. His teachings have been a turning point in my life. My only interest has become to be as close as possible to God."

This Swami is Swami Govind Kaul of Kashmir and I assure the readers that Swamiji had foreseen the entire drama from the time he entered my hutment [hut or camp site] to the moment Dr. Boss got initiated. [He] is said to teach without words, [something] very few people are capable of and Govind Swami is one of them, changing the lives of persons coming into contact with him without preaching. Practice is the soul of realization. He lives in God and teaches others to do so.

J.M. Kayande
(Bharat-Bharati), Goregaon, Bombay[1]

I take away from Kayande's description not only a tribute to Boss, but more important, some details of the encounter between Boss and Kaul that could be transferred to appreciate what happens in the therapeutic setting. At first, "no words were used, no efforts to convince each other."

Boss's conversations with Heidegger on Indian thought preserved in his edition of the Zollikon seminars are relevant here. They are perhaps best represented by the material from their trip to Taormina recorded by Boss. In the section in it on "Sein und Dasein," Boss responds to what Heidegger has just said: "There-being's need to be used as the shepherd [*Hirt*] of the clearing is a distinguished manner of belongingness to the clearing." Boss counters: "Indian thought does not require a shelterer [*Hüter*][2] for the clearing [*Lichtung*]" (663/223/178).

---

1 Kayande's recollection of Boss "prostrating" himself at Kaul's feet is likely a misunderstanding. Boss reports that he was shown yoga postures, which he practiced for the rest of his life. It is probably some such instruction that Kayande had observed.
2 TR gives 'guardian' for *Hüter*.

A. Boss, Heidegger, and the East

Heidegger's formulation here varies from what he had published more than a decade and a half earlier in his *Letter on 'Humanism'* (1947), where he had spoken of *man* [*Mensch*] as the shepherd [*Hirt*] or herdsman of being. At the very beginning of this passage Heidegger had introduced the topic by speaking of man as "the shelterer of the clearing, *of the eventuality* [*Ereignis*]." The meaning for Heidegger of the word 'Ereignis' and how to translate it has been a preoccupation of readers and commentators. The notion's place in his recurring dream may be recalled. I reserve any conclusions about what he means in this passage, but he does *not* say that man is the "guardian of the clearing, of the *disclosive appropriating Event* [of being]" (-/-/178), as we read in *TR*. Perhaps Boss got it wrong in his transcription of their conversations.[1]

This is not the place for a more elaborate reflection on these central ideas from out of Heidegger's thought, but a close reading of this "conversation" (for Trawny, the first minutes) (663-666/223-226/178-181) will be worth the effort.

---

1 In any case, *Hirt* refers to what is watched over (cf. the English word 'herd'), while *Hüter* refers a shepherd's activity watching over [*hütet*] his herd. In the ongoing discussion of be[-]ing (*Sein*) and There-being (*Da-sein*), it is important to keep in mind that *Da-sein* and *Mensch* (man) are not equivalent.

B. From "Da-seinanalysis" to Therapy

My interest in Medard Boss is as the figure who with his existential analysis attempted to bridge psychoanalysis and what is finally emerging as a genuinely human therapy, one not beholden to the medical model. I have presented some till now unknown texts about his personal transformation during the time just before the beginning of the Zollikon seminars and I have tried to bring some clarity to the often bewildering mix of translations of key terms, especially those served by Heidegger's thought.

Boss was unable to complete the transition from psychoanalysis. Standing with one foot steady on the foundational pier built by Freud, he took a broad step to Martin Heidegger's analytics of existence. He straddled two powerful shores and in this bold but somewhat precarious position experienced a personal crisis that has remained for the most part unknown to those of us interested in his existential analysis.

My chief purpose has been to show how and why Boss made genuine therapy possible and to provide some materials—texts, translations and clarifications—that might be used to better understand him and to develop therapy as he envisioned it. I have only hinted at what such therapy might look like, but have independently worked on a version that it may helpful to convey now. It reflects what I think I have learned from Boss, both in what was spoken and published and, more important, what was left unsaid.

Boss's most important paper on practice is "Encounter in Psychotherapy" (1964), which I have recently translated for the first time.

B. From "Da-seinanalysis" to Therapy

Based on what can be found there and drawing on scattered comments he left on practice beginning as early as his book on the paraphilias on through the material from the Zollikon seminars, here is a sketch of what I believe a fully realized therapy grounded in Boss's ideas would look like and how it would be experienced. Until we have access to his *Nachlaß*, we may be allowed some speculation about how he really practiced. I have tried to implement what I take to be Boss's therapeutic prescription in my own practice. What follows are the core elements of that practice which is built on the existential analysis Medard Boss.

The "preverbal understanding... in the present" of the other which Boss spoke of in the last text we examined is a given when any two human beings meet. Being there together or co-existence [*Mit-dasein*] is a given for any human relationship from the earliest years of life. Soon, however, this co-existence is overgrown by a tangle of memories and expectations, most of them social. Much of this mediated by language as it is gradually acquired. We call this enmeshment in the thicket of a culture, which dulls or even occludes co-existence in its open brightness to all that is there, growing up or maturing. That original co-existence disappears in the shadows of a life but it never disappears.

When therapy is in order, the *therapeut* strives to meet in the other what is given *jenseits* to the features of his or her personality. He does this by, to the greatest extent possible, *being nothing in particular* to the other. He is neither doctor nor psychiatrist, neither parent nor teacher. The *therapeut* is already in the present of the other just as the other is in the present of the *therapeut*. This *mutual being already in the present of the other* expresses the notion of co-existence in a different way. It is the preverbal context of anything that follows, which Boss speaks of. An attempt at being nothing to another is difficult to sustain, but it is the craft of therapy.

The second element of therapeutic practice based on Boss's existential analysis is more difficult to describe, and yet it is immediately evident in Boss's experiences with his mentors in India and with Heidegger. It is *taking the other seriously*. This is not necessarily mutual, especially at the beginning of therapy. It may remain unidirectional, from *therapeut* to other, for a long period of time over many meetings.

B. From "Da-seinanalysis" to Therapy

But what does it mean to take someone seriously? And how does one know that he is being taken seriously? This, too, is a preverbal experience and like co-existence is given from the outset in a human life. My understanding of this is based on the assumption that humanness is *not given* but must be passed along during infancy in the primal experience of being taken seriously by the mothering figure. Like co-existence, it is preverbal (*infans* means without speech) and is also marked by our becoming possessed by language, the mother tongue as we call it.

Being taken seriously is being experienced as a *who*, as existing (*Existenz*). It is based on an attunement of one existence with the existence of another. To borrow an image from music, co-existence is "tuned" as the two existing human beings are sound in unison. Anything shy of this amounts to dissonance. It may well be that such dissonance is what we find tried in schizophrenia. To the extent that taking another human being seriously cannot be faked, it cannot be misinterpreted. Its breach is betrayal.

It is my impression that the two sources of what brings a human being to a *therapeut* are not having been taken seriously and the loneliness that is consequent to existential dissonance. While structurally determined by co-existence, as many existential analysts have pointed out, each existence is nevertheless alone. Awareness at some level of this paradox is shared by every living thing and not only human beings. Humans, however, come to know about what they have experienced. Such *Einsamkeit* is the result of our ontological incapacity for understanding the experience of another. Focusing only on behavior is no remedy for this. The paradox of co-existence and *Einsamkeit* is poignant—unspeakable. Much has been written about isolation by "existential-humanistic" psychologists, but I believe they have failed to take into consideration that existence is not equivalent to the human being who embodies it in each case. Nor does realization and acceptance of this or any other commonly named "ultimate concern" lead to improvement. The meaning-making psychotherapies (above all, logotherapy) have addressed these concerns. In each case, however, while claiming to address the existing human being, psychotherapists of such modalities still have in mind some sort of subject. We saw this in the opening dialogue between Längle and Holzhey-Kunz. Genuine

B. From "Da-seinanalysis" to Therapy

therapy, however, is directed only to existence and to the restoration of its present.

Spending time with someone even in the unique therapeutic situation may seem to offer a remedy for our essential solitude, but no remedy is required since there is no ailment. Existing is not subject to the qualifiers healthy or ill. It has been the mistake of psychiatrists following the medical model to make it seem so, however, to generations of well-meaning counselors, psychotherapists, social workers, and other healthcare providers.

Being taken seriously occurs in the context of the way-making concern for the freedom of the other, Boss (following Heidegger) described. Here the particularities of one's body and socioeconomic profile—accidents of genetically transmitted physical features, ethnicity, age, and the rest—are of no importance except as details to be "put in parentheses" (bracketed) to the greatest extent possible. This is the counterpart of the *therapeut's* attempt to be nothing to the other. We may speak of it as taking the other as no one in particular.

What, then, is *the matter* with the other? Nothing. Existence alone is the matter (*Sache*). All particularities add up to a *what*—an identity, a personality, a legal entity, and a body as an ensemble and unity—and so does any diagnosis. Way-making looking after is concerned only with the *who* of existence. Reference to a *what* requires that part of speech we term a noun. Reference to the relative pronoun *who* circumvents that. A who is nameless and without an identity. Precisely ridding existence of this baggage is, of course, the goal of Eastern practices of the kind that attracted Boss first to Hindu philosophy and then to Zen.

We are beholden to what language demands of us but in such a fix, we have abandoned precisely what we wished to preserve and that is the non-reification of existence. If we think of the substantive *Dasein* verbally, however, some of the difficulty disappears. In fact, such a hypothetical verb *dasein* meets the needs of the problematic situation we are attempting to "come to terms with." As such, *dasein* would be a transitive verb. It is my impression that much of Heidegger's deliberation on this term as a substantive in his fundamental ontology only begins to make sense if one considers the sense and use of such a verb in the background of the noun.

B. From "Da-seinanalysis" to Therapy

I experience that I am taken seriously when only my present is of concern to the therapist. This can happen only when nothing I have done (or say or imagine I have done) and nothing I desire or wish for is taken seriously by the therapist.

Conclusion

This is where my reflections on Boss's existential analysis end. I encourage readers to make use of the materials I have assembled to take a fresh look at how Boss may yet affect the direction psychotherapy is to take. His limited influence was due in large part to a lack of clarity in the translations made available to us. This can be remedied. Appreciating something of Boss the man's own struggles also cannot fail to draw us closer to his observations about existential analysis (psychoanalysis without the psyche) and how it must work if it is to have an effect.

The key text, of course, is nothing Boss published under his name. It is the new edition of Martin Heidegger's *Zollikon Seminars* which Boss first edited for publication more than thirty years ago. Without Boss's encouragement and leadership, however, the remarkable meetings of which the book gives an accounting would not have taken place and Boss's existential analysis would not have developed as it did. I have no doubt that there was a special synergy between the two men, who were born only 70 miles apart from each other. They were good for each other at many levels, Heidegger providing Boss with intellectual stimulation that was as meaningful to Boss as his support of Heidegger the man was during the final third of the philosopher's life. This was mutually therapeutic.

Zollikon Seminars is as much Boss's book as it is Heidegger's. It remains the most important document on *Daseinsanalyse*, and any keys to opening the way for a genuinely human therapy are to be found in it. Psychotherapy has possibilities that have not been realized. Boss saw them but got only so far along in realizing them. This is not a failing. We must look at what Boss made possible, keeping in mind what Heidegger said: "Higher than actuality is possibility."

Appendices
Texts and Materials

Appendix I: "Vorwort" to the 2nd Edition of *Sinn und Gehalt der sexuellen Perversionen* (1952)[1]

[7] Das große Interesse, dem dieses Buch in der Welt der wissenschaftlichen Psychologie und Psychopathologie begegnete, und die Bedeutung, die ihm seine Kritiker beimaßen, auferlegten mir die Pflicht, bei der Vorbereitung seiner zweiten Auflage noch einmal alle jene Stellen durchzudenken, deren Formulierung mir nicht unmissverständlich gelungen war. Ich sah mich schließlich vor allem zu zwei Erweiterungen des ursprünglichen Textes gezwungen. Einmal schien es mir dem Verständnis meiner Absichten förderlich zu sein, den bisherigen Entwicklungsweg der Theorien über die sexuellen Perversionen etwas ausführlicher darzustellen. Dadurch hoffte ich noch deutlicher machen zu können, wie dieser Weg von der klassischen psychoanalytischen Psycho-Physik über deren Verwandlung in eine psychoanalytische Ich-Psychologie einerseits und über die Auffassungen der sogenannten anthropologischen Untersucher anderseits zur **daseinsanalytischen** Betrachtungsweise hinführt. Jetzt dürfte gleich von allem Anfang an das schwerwiegende Mißverständnis unmöglich geworden sein, die **daseinsanalytische** Betrachtungsweise bedeute einen Rückfall in eine bloße "Bewußtseins-Psychologie» und stünde der psychoanalytischen,

---

1   In this and the following two appendices, the key terms have been **bolded** for easy reference in studying the translations.

Appendix I

auf unbewußtem Material fußenden Konzeption "feindlich" gegenüber. In Wirklichkeit berücksichtigt die **daseinsanalytische** Betrachtungsweise "das Vorbewußte", und "das Unbewußte" nicht weniger als alles vom Kranken bereits Gewußte. Gerade deshalb vermag sie aber auch alle früheren Einsichten in sich aufzunehmen und eine diese als Teilaspekte tragende Verstehensbasis zu bilden.

Nun sollte auch der Umstand, daß mehr und mehr die gewohnte psychoanalytische Terminologie vermieden wurde, nicht mehr länger diesem Mißverständnis Vorschub leisten. Denn die offenere, vorsichtigere **daseinsanalytische** Ausdrucksweise wurde nur darum bevozugt, weil die psychoanalytische *Theorie* mit ihren abstrakten Begriffen eines "Es", eines "Ichs", eines "Überichs" usw. nur allzu leicht zu einer gefährlichen Versachlichung, Vergegenständlichung und künstlichen Zerstückelung des Menschen verführt. Die klassische psychoanalytische *Praxis* und Technik freilich wird von [8] diesen Einwänden überhaupt nicht berührt. Sie hat sich auch mir stets als das unübertreffliche Verfahren bewährt, um meinen Kranken die von ihnen zunächst regelmäßig nicht gewußten, pathologisch verstimmten, ihre Welt- und Selbsterfahrungen je und je bestimmenden Grundbefindlichkeiten greifbar und damit auch therapeutisch angreifbar zu machen. Ich erweiterte ferner im ersten Teil des Buches den Abschnitt über die "Psychologischen Bemerkungen zur Norm der Liebe". Ich versuchte dabei, die Phänomene des Liebens noch ursprünglicher auf die fundamentalen Wesensstrukturen des **menschlichen Daseins** zu beziehen, so wie sie uns *Martin Heidegger* aufgezeigt hat. Je tiefer die Einsichten in das Wesen des menschlichen Liebens überhaupt zu dringen vermögen, um so weiter öffnet sich auch der Verstehenshorizont für die Phänomene der sexuellen Perversionen.

Den zweiten Teil des Buches, in dem die konkreten Einzelschicksale sexuell perverser Menschen beschrieben werden, durfte ich im großen und ganzen unverändert lassen. Alle die sexuell perversen Kranken, in deren Lebensgeschichte mich die psychoanalytische Praxis seit der Publikation der ersten Auflage noch hatte Einblick gewinnen lassen, haben mir nur immer wieder die volle Bestätigung dieser Darstellungen gebracht.

Zürich, im Frühjahr 1951. *M. Boss.*

Appendix II: "Vorwort" to the 3rd Edition of *Sinn und Gehalt der sexuellen Perversionen* (1966)

[9] Seit den Tagen, da die vorliegende Schrift zum erstenmal in den Druck ging, sind zwanzig Jahre vergangen. Im Verlauf dieser langen Zeit sind dem Autor noch Dutzende von neuen Kranken, die an sexuellen Perversionen litten, zu Gesicht gekommen. Einige von ihnen hatte er selbst zu behandeln; der größte Teil waren Kranke, deren Therapie von seinen Schülern durchgeführt wurde, alle aber unter seiner ständigen Kontrolle.

Keine einzige dieser weiteren zwanzigjährigen Erfahrungen widersprach in irgend einer grundsätzlichen Weise dem schon in der ersten Auflage dieses Buches beschriebenen Sinn und Gehalt der sexuellen Perversionen. Darin darf füglich ein überzeugender Beleg mehr für die Stichhaltigkeit der damals gewonnenen Einsichten erblickt werden.

Andererseits würde es für eine unverzeihliche geistige Trägheit des Autors zeugen, wären ihm in der Zwischenzeit nicht eine noch zutreffendere gedankliche Fassung und klarere Fundierung der vor zwei Jahrzehnten erblickten Sachverhalte möglich geworden. "Sinn und Gehalt der sexuellen Perversionen" entstand ja als eine allererste Frucht der Berührung meiner ärztlich-psychiatrischen Erfahrungen mit dem neuen Menschenverständnis, das wir der philosophischen **Daseinsanalytik** Martin Heideggers zu verdanken haben. Diese nun schon drei Jahrzehnte dauernde Auseinandersetzung der Psychiatrie mit der **Daseinsanalytik** war aber besonders an ihrem Beginn durch einige grundlegende und überaus verwirrende Mißverständnisse von Seiten der Ärzte gekennzeichnet.

Schuld an diesen Mißverständnissen war vor allem das Nachwirken der "Phänomenologie" Husserls bei den ärztlichen Vertretern der neu aufkommenden "psychiatrischen **Daseinsanalytik**". Husserls "Phänomenologie" aber ist eine solche des Ich-Bewußtseins und bleibt damit der Vorstellung vom Menschen als einer Subjektivität verhaftet. Dagegen legt der alles bestimmende Entwurf des Menschseins als "**Dasein**", [10] wie ihn Heidegger in seiner **Daseinsanalytik** herauskristallisierte, in schärfstem Gegensatz dazu alles darauf an, diese subjektivistische Vorstellung zu sprengen; besser: gar nicht erst aufkommen zu lassen.

Schuld an den verwirrenden Mißverständnissen der frühen "**daseinsanalytischen**" Psychiater war ferner deren ständige Verkennung der ontologischen Bestimmungen des Menschseins in der **Daseinsanalytik** Heideggers als ontische Feststellungen am menschlichen Verhalten. Aus solcher Verwechslung erwuchs die Unmöglichkeit eines geklärten Verständnisses für das Verhältnis zwischen wesenhafter, ontologischer Aussage über das Menschsein und den ontisch-psychiatrisch feststellbaren menschlichen Phänomenen.

Glücklicherweise erfolgte die notwendige Klärung dieser psychiatrischen Verwirrung in den letzten Jahren zugleich von den beiden einzig maßgeblichen Seiten her. Einmal wagte 1958 Ludwig Binswanger, dem das bleibende Verdienst zukommt, als erster die Psychiater auf das epochemachende Werk Martin Heideggers aufmerksam gemacht zu haben, das überaus mutige öffentliche Eingeständnis, er habe in der Tat Heidegger Denken mißverstanden. Folgerichtig ließ Binswanger seither auch immer konsequenter die seinerzeit aus Heideggers Werk "Sein und Zeit" übernommenen Bezeichnungen "**Daseinsanalyse**" und "**daseinsanalytisch**" als Titel für seine eigenen Arbeiten fallen und bezog sich von da an nur mehr auf Husserls "Phänomenologie". Durch diesen seltenen wissenschaftlichen und menschlichen Mut gebot Binswanger nach Möglichkeit dem

Appendix II

Weiterwuchern des gedanklichen Durcheinanders Einhalt, das namentlich bei den Lernenden deshalb zustande kommen mußte, weil anfänglich gleichlautende Titel für zwei völlig voneinander verschiedene Auffassungen vom Grundwesen des Menschen verwendet wurden.

Zum andern kommen seit rund fünf Jahren die angehenden Zürcher Psychiater in den Genuß regelmäßiger Seminarien, die Heidegger selbst zwei- bis dreimal im Semester in [11] Zusammenarbeit mit dem Autor dieser Schrift in Zollikon Zürich abhält. Bei diesen Gelegenheiten wird auch Heidegger nicht müde, den Psychiatern zu bestätigen, daß von Ludwig Binswanger in die Psychiatrie eingeführte Vorstelle mit seinem **daseinsanalytischen** Verständnis zu tun habe. Es könne vielmehr gar keinen größeren Irrtum geben als den, Binswanger mit seiner Charakterisierung der **Daseinsanalytischen** Verständnis als einer äußerst konsequenten Fortsetzung der Lehre Kant und Husserl begangen habe.

So ist denn von den beiden kompetentesten Stellen her mit aller wünschenswerten Deutlichkeit klargestellt worden, welche Art von psychiatrischer Arbeit überhaupt etwas mit Heideggers **Daseinsanalytik** und seinen einzelnen **Daseinsanalysen** zu tun hat und welche nicht mit seiner Sicht in Zusammenhang gebracht werden können, denen deshalb auch der Titel "**daseinsanalytisch**" von der Sache her nicht zusteht, weil er seinem Schöpfer für eine ganz andere Denk- und Schweise erfunden wurde.

Weil hierüber nun kein Zweifel mehr möglich ist, steht zu erwarten, daß dem vorbildlichen Vorgehen L. Binswangers bald auch dessen zögernde Schuler nachfolgen werden. Auch sie werden demnächst ihre wissenschaftlich Arbeitsweise nicht länger eine »**daseinsanalytische**« nennen wollen, sondern werden sie einen anderen Namen zu finden suchen.

Eine reinliche, auch nomenklatorisch festgemachte Scheidung vom **daseinsanalytischen** Zugang zu den psychopathologischen Phänomenen kann ihnen schon deshalb nicht schwer fallen, mit einem solch offenen Zugeständnis der Andersartigtkeit ihrer Untersuchungsmethode gegenüber jener von Heideggers **Daseinsanalytik** und den faktisch in dieser gründen psychiatrischen **Daseinsanalysen** noch nicht das geringste über einen möglichen qualitativen Unterschied in

Appendix II

der Angemessenheit der einen und anderen Sicht an die Sache der Psychiatrie hinsichtlich ihrer Fruchtbarkeit für diese präjudiziert.

An den bedeutsamen Ereignissen, die sich im Laufe des [12] vergangenen Jahrzehnts aus dem Gebiete der Psychiatrie abspielten, durfte selbstverständlich auch die Vorbereitung der dritten Auflage von "Sinn und Gehalt der sexuellen Perversionen" nicht achtlos vorbeigeben, lief doch Heidegger persönliche, fortlaufende Auseinandersetzung mit der psychiatrischen Disziplin eine für diese entscheidende Differenzierung zwischen zwei grundlegenden Sachverhalten mit früher nicht gekannter Präzision vollziehen. Es kann jetzt klarer als zuvor die philosophisch-ontologische **Daseinsanalytik** und deren Vollzug in Gestalt der einzelnen ontologischen **Daseinsanalysen**, wie sie in "Sein und Zeit" erarbeitet worden waren, von einer **ontisch-daseinsanalytischen** Psychopathologie und deren Vollzug in Beschreibungen und Interpretationen konkreter, psychiatrisch feststellbarer menschlicher Verhaltensweisen unterschieden werden, die sich als solche im Horizont jener philosophisch-ontologiscben **Daseinsanalytik** und **Daseinsanalyse** bewegen.

Alle diese grundlegenden Klärungen hinsichtlich des Verhältnisses zwischen Philosophie und Psychiatrie machten eine wesentliche Umarbeitung der ersten Kapitel des vorliegenden Buches unumgänglich, zielen diese doch auf eine Wesensbestimmung des normgemäßen menschlichen Liebenkönnens ab. Eine solch grundlegende Besinnung war von Anfang an unerläßlich, sollten die folgenden Abschnitte, die die psychopathologischen Liebesphänomene behandeln, nicht in der Luft hängen bleiben, sondern auf einem tragenden Grund und Boden zu stehen kommen. Alles krankhafte Verhalten ist ja immer nur sachgemäß als eine Privationserscheinung der normgemäßen Beziehungsmöglichkeiten, also als ein Mangel an Gesundheit zu begreifen. Als Privationsphänomen, als ein Mangelzustand an Gesundheit bleibt alles Krankhafte stets und notwendigerweise auf das normgemäße, gesunde Menschsein als seine Basis bezogen. Das normgemäße Liebenkönnen seinerseits ist immer nur eine der möglichen Vollzugsweisen des Menschseins im ganzen. Darum ist für ein rechtes Begreifen des normgemäßen wie auch allen pathologischen Liebesverhaltens [13] eine Einsicht in die Wesenszüge, in die spezifische Seinsart, die Grundnatur des Men-

Appendix II

schseins im ganzen die unabdingbare Voraussetzung. Man hat sich, mit anderen Worten, auch bei aller psychologisch-psychiatrischen Forschung stets vorgängig in bezug auf eine zureichende ontologische Bestimmungen ins klare zu bringen. Alles faktisch feststellbare menschliche Verhalten wird von den in den ontologischen Bestimmungen artikulierten Wesenszügen des Menschseins als von seinem Eigensten schon immer und ständig durchwaltet. Deshalb darf nie die bequeme Rede davon sein, das ontologische Denken vom ontisch-psychiatrischen Beobachten und Interpretieren trennen und jenes ganz den Philosophen überlassen zu wollen.

Freilich ist und bleibt stets die eigentliche Ausarbeitung und Sichtbarmachung der ontologischen Bestimmungen des Menschseins die Aufgabe der wesentlichen Denker, der Philosophen und kann nie das Geschäft der ärztlichen Psychopathologen oder der wissenschaftlichen Psychologen sein. Aus diese grundlegende Vorarbeit der Denker sind deshalb alle Psychologen und Psychiater, auch alle Sexualpathologen angewiesen. Es zeugt von einer in ihrer Oberflächligkeit überaus gefährlichen Verkennung der eigenen Möglichkeiten psychologischer und psychiatrischer Autoren, wenn immer wieder einer psychiatrischen Betrachtungsweise daraus ein Vorwurf gemacht wird, das sie sich streng im Horizonte von Wesenseinsichten bewegt, die sie dem Denken eines Philosophen verdankt.

Im Bereiche der dem allgemeinen Teil des Buches folgenden Darstellung von acht konkreten Krankengeschichten sexuell perverser Menschen waren indessen auf Grund der Neubearbeitung der Einführungskapitel verhältnismäßig wenige Änderungen vonnöten. Immerhin sind auch die Neuformulierungen hier einschneidend genug, um erhoffen zu lassen, das sie ebenfalls mithelfen werden, den Sinn und Gehalt der sexuellen Perversionen, wie sie den Kranken selbst abgelauscht und ihrer wesentlichen Bedeutung nach schon in der ersten Auflage dargestellt worden waren, jetzt noch viel reiner und plastischer hervortreten zu lassen.

Im August 1966. MEDARD Boss

Appendix III: "Nachwort" to the 3rd Edition of *Sinn und Gehalt der sexuellen Perversionen* (1966)

[174] Nicht lange nach dem Erscheinen der 2. Auflage der vorstehenden Schrift hatte der entschiedenste Verrreter der sogenannten "anthropologischen Perversions-Theorie", v. Gebsattel, unsere Kritik an seiner Auffassung eines eigenen Entgegnungs-Kapitels in seinen 1954 erschienenen "Prolegomena einer medizinischen Anthropologie" gewürdigt. Mit Scharfblick erkannte er dort, daß "der Streit um die Richtigkeit **daseinsanalytischen** oder der anthropologischen Theorie genauer der um den *Symbolwert* der in ihrer Sonderstruktur voll erfaßten oder nicht voll erfaßten perversen Akte" sei (Seite 218).

[175] Mit nichts anderem jedoch als mit diesem "Argument", das einen in den perversen Akten angeblich enthaltenen *Symbolwert* über die Richtigkeit oder Unrichtigkeit seiner Auffassung entscheiden lassen will, hatte v. Gebsattel schlagender beweisen können, wie wenig er sich bei seiner Theorie an die von den Kranken erfahrenen Phänomene selbst und an die diesen wesensmäßig zugehörigen und sie recht eigentlich ausmachenden Bedeutungsgehalte und Verweisungszusammenhänge hält. Denn was ist der sogenannte *Symbolwert* einer Sache je anderes als jener intellektuell-emotionale Gehalt, den der Betrachter der sogenannten reinen Tatsachlichkeit eines

Appendix III

Phänomens noch zusätzlich von sich aus und aus seiner "unbewußten Psyche" heraus 'psychologisch" zuschreibt und hinzufügt? In einem derartigen "symbolischen" Vorgehen läßt sich die ganze unüberbrückbare Kluft zwischen allen subjektivistisch-anthropologischen Theorien und der besonderen Zugangsart einer **daseinsanalytisch-phänomenologischen** Menschenkunde mit Händen greifen. Nichts aber ist vorzüglicher dazu geeignet, die **daseinsanalytisch-phänomenologische** Untersuchungsmethode, die die vorliegende Schrift überhaupt erst möglich machte, sich ständig durchwaltet und in allen Einzelheiten bestimmt, in ihr eigenes Wesen einzugrenzen und sie als das, was sie ist und sein will, zum Vorschein kommen zu lassen, als ein Deutlichmachen gerade dieser Kluft, die sie von allen "anthropologischen" Theorien trennt. Darum sei als Erstes die Kennzeichnung sogenannter symbolischer Werte und Gehalte angeführt, wie wir sie M. Heidegger verdanken.

In seinem Aufsatz "Bauen, Wohnen, Denken" beschreibt Heidegger, um an einem Beispiel den einem Ding selbst zugehörigen Reichtum an Bedeutungsgehalten sichtbar werden zu lassen, eine Brücke. Er erwähnt dabei u. a.: "Die Brücke schwingt sich, 'leicht und kräftig', über den Strom. Sie verbindet nicht nur schon vorhandene Ufer. Im Übergang der Brücke treten die Ufer erst als Ufer hervor. Die Brücke läßt sie eigens gegeneinander über liegen. Die andere Seite [176] ist durch die Brücke gegen die eine abgesetzt. Die Ufer ziehen auch nicht als gleichgültige Grenzstreifen des festen Landes den Strom entlang. Die Brücke bringt mit den Ufern jeweils die eine und die andere Weite der rückwärtigen Uferlandschaft an den Strom. Sie bringt Strom und Ufer und Lund in die wechselseitige Nachbarschaft. Die Brücke *versammelt* die Erde als Landschaft um den Strom. So geleitet sie ihn durch die Auen. Die Brückenpfeiler tragen, aufruhend im Strombett, den Schwung der Bogen, die den Wassern des Stromes ihre Bahn lassen ... Die Brücke läßt dem Strom seine Bahn und gewährt zugleich den Sterblichen ihren Weg, daß sie von Land zu Land gehen und fahren. Brücken geleiten auf mannigfache Weise. Die Stadtbrücke fuhrt vom Schloßbezirk zum Domplatz, die Flußbrücke vor der Landstadt bringt Wagen und Gespann zu den umliegenden Dörfern. Der unscheinbare Bachübergang der alten Steinbrücke gibt dem Erntewagen seinen Weg von der Flur in das Dorf, trägt die Holzfuhre vom Feldweg zur

Appendix III

Landstraße. Die Autobahnbrücke ist eingespannt in das Liniennetz des rechnenden und möglichst schnellen Fernverkehrs. Immer und je anders geleitet die Brücke hin und her die zögernden und die hastigen Wege der Menschen, das sie zu anderen Ufern und zuletzt als die Sterblichen auf die andere Seite kommen. Die Brücke überschwingt bald auf hohen, bald in flachen Bogen Fluß und Schlucht; ob die Sterblichen das Überschwingende der Brückenbahn in der Acht behalten oder vergessen, daß sie, immer schon unterwegs zur letzten Brücke, im Grunde danach trachten, ihr Gewöhnliches und Unheiles zu übersteigen, um sich vor das Heile des Göttlichen zu bringen. Die Brücke *sammelt* als der überschwingende Übergang vor die Göttlichen. Mag deren Anwesen eigens bedacht und sichtbarlich bedankt sein wie in der Figur des Brückenheiligen, mag es verstellt oder gar weggeschoben bleiben."

Nach solcher Erfassung der Brücke in ihrem eigenen und vollen Bedeutungs- und Verweisungszusammenhang ist es für [177] Heidegger ein Leichtes, den "symbolischen" Irrtum der heute geläufigen Psychologien zu korrigieren. Er fährt an der nämlichen Stelle fort: "Man meint freilich, die Brücke sei zunächst und eigentlich *bloß* eine Brücke. Nachträglich und gelegentlich könne sie dann auch noch mancherlei ausdrücken. Als ein solcher Ausdruck werde sie dann zum Symbol, zum Beispiel für all das, was vorhin genannt wurde. Allein die Brücke ist, wenn sie eine echte Brücke ist, niemals zuerst bloße Brücke und hinterher ein Symbol in dem Sinn, daß sie etwas ausdrückt, was, streng genommen, nicht zu ihr gehört. Wenn wir die Brücke streng nehmen, zeigt sie sich nie als Ausdruck. Die Brücke ist ein Ding und *nur dies* ... Unser Denken ist freilich von altersher gewohnt, das Wesen des Dinges *zu dürftig* anzusetzen. Dies hat im Verlauf des abendländischen Denkens zur Folge, daß man das Ding als ein unbekanntes X vorstellt, das mit wahrnehmbaren Eigenschaften behaftet ist. Von da aus gesehen erscheint uns freilich alles, *was schon zum versammelnden Wesen dieses Dinges gehört*, als nachträglich hineingedeutete Zutat".[1]

---

1 M. Heidegger, Vorträge und Aufsätze, 1954, 153 ff. Zur Kritik am psychologischen Symbolbegriff siehe ferner: M. Boss, Der Traum und seine Auslegung, 1953, 96 ff.

Appendix III

Grundsätzlich genau so wie bei den "psychologischen Symbolisierungen" einer Brücke entspringt auch das Suchen nach dem 'Symbolwert', der nach Meinung anthropologischer Psychopathologen von den sexuell perversen Menschen ihrem geschlechtlichen Verhalten geheimerweise zugelegt werden soll, dem zu dürftigen Ansetzen des Wesens eben dieses Verhaltens selbst. Lassen wir dieses nur immer selbst durch den Mund der Kranken zu uns sprechen, kündet es uns seinem eigenen grundlegenden Wesen nach -- wie alles sexuelle Verhalten überhaupt -- nie von Nihilismus und Zerstörung, sondern stets von Weitung, Einung, Mehrung, von Überwindung alltäglicher Konturen.

An zweiter Stelle dürfen wir uns damit begnügen, auf [178] jene Ausführungen von G. Condrau zu verweisen, durch die uns dieser Auter die Kritik an der Kritik von v. Gebsattel bereits 1965 vorweg und abgenommen hat.[1]

Condrau schreibt, unseres Erachtens mit vollem Recht, "In gewisser Weise näher als Kunz steht der **Daseinsanalyse** von Boss der "anthropologische" Psychiater V. E. v. Gebsattel. Allerdings hat auch er manches an der **daseinsanalytischen** Betrachtungsweise auszusetzen. Seine Kritik richtet sich ins besondere gegen das **daseinsanalytische** Verstehen des Wesens und des Sinngehaltes der sexuellen Perversionen. In diesem Bereiche erscheint ihm "eine Revision der **daseinsanalytischen** Theorie ... geboten".[2] Wenn Boss auch noch in den perversen Kümmer- und Verstümmelungsformen, meint v. Gebsattel ferner, eine eindeutige Manifestation der Liebe sehe, so mute diese Einschätzung von Geschlechtsverkehr und Orgasmus naiv an und repräsentiere fraglos den schwachen Punkt der neuen, **daseinsanalytischen** Perversionstheorie.[3]

Der naiv geheißenen Qualifizierung von Boss stellt v. Gebsattel seine eigene "anthropologische" Deutung entgegen, die in allen sexuellen perversen Akten den *"Zug und Hang zum Bösen* -- oder wenn wir in einer anthropologischen Betrachtungsweise diese moral-theologisch klingende Wendung vermeiden wollen -- *den nihilistischen Grundzug*

---

1 G. Condrau, Die Daseinsanalyse von Medard Boß und ihre Bedeutung für die Psychiatrie, 1965, 80 ff.
2 V. Gebsattel, Prolegomena einer medizinischen Anthropologie, 1954, 220.
3 Loc. cit., 217.

der menschlichen Natur" erkennen will. Boss wird vorgeworfen, er über sehe einfach, daß es im Menschen auch "eine libidinöse Lust am Zerstören, an der Destruktion als solcher" gebe und daß sich diese überall in den sexuellen Perversionen symbolisch zum Ausdruck bringe.[1]

Ganz so fraglos, wie es sich v. Gebsattel wünscht, wird indessen kaum ein Kenner der Sache diese Behauptung des Kritikers übernehmen. "Naiv" wird sich Boss freilich gerne [179] nennen lassen, wenn v. Gebsattel darunter eine Betrachtungsweise versteht, die bei den Bedeutungsgehalten und Verweisungszusammenhängen der einem Menschen begegnenden Phänomene verweilen will, so wie sie sich von diesen selbst her unversehrt und unmittelbar zeigen und vernehmen lassen. Bei diesem seinem Bemühen um einen phänomenologischen Zugang zu den Dingen weiß sich nämlich Boss frei von der Schuld an der durch keine ausweisbaren Momente gerechtfertigten Degradierung des Betrachteten zu etwas Uneigentlichem, bloß "symbolisch" Ausgedrücktem, wie es notwendigerweise der "anthropologischen" Deutung v. Gebsattels innewohnt. Denn indem v. Gebsattel nach einem hintergründigen "Symbolwert" der sexuell perversen Akte fragt, läßt er diese zum vorneherein immer zu etwas nur noch Abgeleitetem werden, abgeleitet eben von irgendwelchen hinter den Phänomenen angenommenen, ihnen unterstellten, aus ihnen nur gedanklich erschlossenen Strebungen, "Zügen" und "Hängen". Wo immer jedoch zwischen zwei Sachen ein der artiges Ausdrucksverhältnis hineingedacht wird, bleibt seiner eigentlichen Natur nach sowohl das Sichausdrückende wie Ausgedrückte dunkel.[2]

Die "naive", unmittelbare Selbsterfahrung aller bisher von Boss und seinen Schülern wahrend Monaten und Jahren psychoanalytisch beobachteten sexuell perversen Menschen hat aber ausnahmslos weder die Patienten selbst noch ihre Analytiker je einen urständigen "Hang zum Bösen" oder einen "nihilistischen Grundzug der menschlichen Natur" in Zusammenhang mit dem krankhaften Verhalten direkt erkennen lassen. Vielmehr wurde auch von diesen Kranken das sexuelle Erleben bis hinauf zum Orgasmus stets und ausschließlich innerhalb des Bedeutungsgehaltes eines Überwindens von Schranken,

---

1 Loc. cit, 219.
2 Vgl. M. Boss, Einführung in die psychosomatische Medizin, 1954, 87.

Appendix III

eines "Über-sich-selbst-hinaus" erfahren, wenn ihnen dabei ebenso ausnahmslos auch noch so vieles an erlösender [180] Befreiung und Weitung fehlte, die einem normgemäßen Liebesakt innezuwohnen pflegt. Dies aber heißt mit anderen Worten, daß jeder einzelne perverse Sexualakt keineswegs etwas qualitativ ganz anderes als ein normgemäßes Lieben ist, sondern lediglich dessen *privative* Erscheinung darstellt. Eine Privation aber ist grundsätzlich alles andere als die Verneinung dessen, dem etwas 'geraubt' wurde, dem etwas fehlt. Schon gar nicht wird zufolge einer Privation ein Phänomen in seinem Sinn und Gehalt in sein Gegenteil verkehrt. Vielmehr verweist jedes privative Phänomen erst recht auf den vollen Bedeutungsgehalt der unversehrten Erscheinung. So ist jeder Schatten zum Beispiel durchaus nicht das Gegenteil von Helle. Dem Schatten fehlt nur etwas an Helle. Gerade dank dieses seines privativen Charakterzuges gehört deshalb auch jeder Schatten in den Bedeutungsgehalt "Helligkeit" hinein.

Wenn v. Gebsattel die überaus sorgfältigen konkreten Krankenbeobachtungen von Boss dadurch entwerten will, daß er die dargestellten Fälle als nicht voll perverse, nicht voll triebanormale Psychopathen bezeichnet, ist dieser Einwand leicht abzuwehren. Mit Ausnahme von zwei seiner angeführten sexuell perversen Kranken waren nämlich alle übrigen von berufener klinisch-psychiatrischer Seite als voll triebanormale Psychopathen klassifiziert worden. Soll deshalb dieser Einwand v. Gebsattels von Gewicht werden, muß der Kritiker schon konkrete Krankengeschichten gleich sorgfältig untersuchter sexuell Perverser vorlegen, deren Selbsterfahrung die von v. Gebsattel erschlossene "Symboldeutung" unmittelbar erkennen lassen.

Bisher jedoch finden wir in v. Gebsattels Kritik anstelle konkreter, direkter Belege in Form von Selbsterfahrungen sexuell perverser Menschen nur die Behauptung, es bedürfe eben zur Annahme seiner »anthropologischen Perversionstheorie" [181] des "Standpunktes einer Anthropologie", die das Bild des Menschen anderen Kategorien unterstellt als den von Boss entwickelten.

Die Stichhaltigkeit dieses zweiten "Argumentes" gegen das **daseinsanalytische** Verstehen der sexuellen Perversionen bedenkt man mit Vorteil auf Grund jener Ausführungen Heideggers über das Wesen der neuzeitlichen Anthropologien ganz im allgemeinen, die im

Aufsatz »"Die Zeit des Weltbildes" zu lesen sind.[1] Sie beginnen mit dem Hinweis darauf, daß in allen heutigen Anthropologien jene philosophische Deutung des Menschen geschehe, die vom Menschen aus und auf den Menschen zu das Seiende im Ganzen erkläre und abschätze. Diese Kennzeichnung wird später noch folgendermaßen erläutert: "Anthropologie ist jene Deutung des Menschen, die ja im Grunde schon weiß, was der Mensch ist und daher nie fragen kann, wer er sei. Denn mit dieser Frage müßte sie sich selbst als erschüttert und überwunden bekennen. Wie soll dies der Anthropologie zugemutet werden, wo sie doch eigens und nur die nachträgliche Sicherung der Selbstsicherheit des Subjectum zu leisten hat?"

In der Tat weiß auch v. Gebsattel schon zum vornherein, daß der Mensch einen primären Zug und Hang zum Bösen, zum Sündigen und zum Nichts besitzt und daß ihm die Befriedigung dieser destruktiven Bedürfnisse ebenso wie die der erotischen Strebungen eine "libidinöse Lust" zu bringen vermag. Würde nämlich die Anthropologie und Moraltheologie v. Gebsattels dies alles nicht schon voraussetzen, könnte er gewiß nicht seine Kritik an Boss durch die Anekdote krönen und ihr gar die Schlüsselgewalt zum Aufschließen des Geheimnisses der sexuellen Perversionen zutrauen, die im Folgenden wiedergegeben sei. Sie stammt -- so vermutet v. Gebsattel -- nicht von ungefähr aus den Kreisen des letzten großen französischen Pessimisten und Moralisten Chamfort [182] der 1794 Suizid beging. Er referiert sie folgendermaßen: "Es handelt sich um eine liebenswürdige, aber wohl irgendwie leicht verderbte, junge Dame. Sie verschafft sich in einer heißen Gegend - sagen wir Neapel - den Genuß eines Fruchteises. Ein Seufzer entringt sich ihr beim Schlürfen der Kühlung spendenden Speise, aber zu diesem Seufzer bewegt sie nicht der unmittelbare Genuß, sondern seinen eigentlichen Sinn verrät ihr Ausruf: "Ah! Quel dommage, ce n'est pas un peche." "Also", schließt v. Gebsattel sogleich daraus, "der Kühlung spendenden Köstlichkeit fehlt etwas, um zum Vollgenuß zu werden; etwas entbehrt unsere junge Freundin offenbar; den sündigen Einschlag nämlich ihres Genusses; dieser erst, dieses moralische oder besser: unmoralische Element, mittels dessen die sinnliche Unmittelbarkeit der Welteinung überstiegen würde,

---

1 M. Heidegger, *Holzwege*, 1950, pp. 86 and 103.

Appendix III

wäre erst, so bekundet ihr Seufzer, des sinnlichen Genusses eigentliche Würze".[1]

Wie aber, wenn diese junge Dame gar nicht so verderbe und unmoralisch, wenn sie nur ein besonders lebensvolles Mädchen gewesen wäre? Wie, wenn beim Eis-Essen das Fehlen vitalitätshemmender, pseudo-moralischer Sünden-Schranken Schuld an dem Mangel an Genuß gehabt hätte, und zwar deshalb, weil damit auch die Möglichkeit eines Überwindens und Durchbrechens solcher Schranken fehlte? Wir wissen ja zur Genüge, daß eine ganze Menge bigottester Prüderie-Schranken das Leben der damaligen jungen Mädchen eingekehrt hielt. Mit welchem Recht würde dann aber v. Gebsattel die Lust nach einem Übersteigen und Durchbrechen solcher Fesseln einen Hang zum Bösen, zur Destruktion und zum Nichts heißen dürfen? Konnte dieses Mädchens Wunsch nach "Sündigen«" nicht viel angemessener denn als "Nihilismus" als eine unmittelbar lustvolle Bewegung gerade auf "Welteinung", auf Selbstbefreiung und auf Zulassen konventionell verbotener, aber ihrem eigensten Wesen zugehöriger Lebensrnöglichkeiten hin verstanden werden?

---

1 von Gebsattel, *loc. cit.*, 220.

Appendix IV: A Comparison of the Table of Contents of the First (1947) and Second (1952) Editions of *Sinn und Gehalt der sexuellen Perversionen*

The Two Editions

The organization of the two editions is the same. The TOC of the first edition is given and the one change is chapter title is noted.

Table of Contents

I   Einleitung
II Die psychoanalytische Perversionstheorie
III Zur Kritik der psychoanalytischen Perversionstheorie
IV Die 'anthroplogischen' Perversionstheorie
VI Psychologischen Bemerkungen zur Norm der Liebe

Appendix IV

VII Die Dialektik von Liebe und 'Welt' und ihre Störungen bei sexuell perversen Menschen[1]
    A   Ein Fetischist
    B   Ein Koprophiler
    C   Eine Kleptomanin
    D   Ein Voyeur und Exhibitionist
    E   Ein Sado-Masochist
    F   Drei Homosexuelle
        1   Eine psychoneurotische Homosexuelle
        2   Ein psychotischer Homosexueller
        3   Eine 'konstitutionell' Homosexuelle
VIII Schluß

A notable change is found when Boss distinguishes his *Daseinsanalyse* from Binswanger's:

First Edition: "In order to differentiate our way of considering things from the earlier anthropological research approach and terminology, with L. Binswanger we prefer the expression 'existential analysis'. For with 'love' and 'world' we really intend to include the whole existence of man."[2]

Second Edition: "In order to differentiate our way of considering things from both the views of classic psychoanalysis as well as from the terminology of the previous 'anthropological' research approach, we prefer the Heideggerian term analytics of existence."[3]

---

1 "The Dialectics of Love and 'World' and Their Disturbances in Sexually Perverse Human Beings." In SG²: "Die Beinträchtigungen der normgemäßen Verwirklichungsmöglichkeiten der Liebe bei sexuell perversen Menschen [The Impairments of Normative Possibilities of Fulfillment of Love in Sexually Perverse Human Beings]."
2 Um dabei unsere Betrachtungsweise sowohl von der bisherigen anthropologischen Forschungsrichtung auch terminologisch zu unterscheiden, ziehen wir für sie mit L. Binswanger den Ausdruck 'Daseinsanalyse' vor. Denn wir meinen, mit 'Liebe' und 'Welt' wirklich das ganze Dasein des Menschen einbezogen zu haben. SG1 34.
3 Um dabei unsere Betrachtungsweise sowohl von den Anschauungen der klassischen psychoanalytischen Theorie wie von der bisherigen 'anthropo-

Appendix IV

References to Heidegger

There are a number of references to Heidegger in the two editions. These are given by page number for the two editions:

First Edition: SG[1]

18 In modern philosophy, following on Husserl's phenomenology this fundamental question about 'being' was introduced by Heidegger.[1]
28 [fundamental ontology (*Fundamentalontologie*)] [anxious care (*ängstlichen Sorge*)]
29 [note 7]
32 [care (*Sorge*)]
40 ... the existential-analytical approach means anxiety is a primary 'basic condition' of existence in general (Heidegger), indeed of human existence in precisely its world-isolated way of ek-sisting.[2]
41 However, Freud (and this is his special merit) has grasped with these two 'complexes' [dread of incest, fear of castration] very significant breaches of this existensive anxiety, in which existence is always anxious both *in the face of* and *about* its being in the world.[3]
42 Anxiety, however, is the characteristic fundamental temperament (Heidegger) and at the same time most significant barrier of the world isolated, ultimately finite, purposefully restricted form of existing.[4]

---

logischen' Forschungsrichtung auch terminologisch zu unterscheiden, ziehen wir für sie den Heideggerschen Namen 'Daseinsanalytik' vor. SG[2] 40.

1 In die Philosophie der Neuzeit wurde diese Fundamentalfrage nach dem 'Sein' im Anschluß an Husserls Phänomenologie durch Martin Heidegger [SZ] eingeführt.
2 ... der daseinsanalytischen Betrachtungsweise bedeutet vielmehr die Angst eine primäre 'Grundbefindlichkiet' des Daseins (Heidegger) überhaupt, und zwar des menschlichen Daseins eben in der Weise weltlich-isolierten Existieren-müssens.
3 Allerdings hat Freud, und das ist sein besonderes Verdienst, mit diesen beiden 'Komplexen' [Inzestscheu, Kastrationsfurcht] sehr bedeutsame Einbruchstellen dieser Existenzialangst erfaßt, in der sich Dasein immer ängstigt *vor* und *um* sein In-der-Welt-sein zugleich (Heidegger SZ 187).
4 Angst aber ist die kennzeichende Grundstimmung (Heidegger) und zugleich die bedeutsamste Schranke der weltlich isolierten, endlich begrenzten, zweckhaft eingeengsten Existenzform.

Appendix IV

123 Seeing through the abstract character of psychoanalytic theory, the so-called anthropological psychopathologists believed that they had gotten their impetus mainly from Jaspers, E. Minkowski, and Heidegger....[1]

124 ['care' (Heidegger) ('*Sorge*' (Heidegger))]

Second Edition: SG[2]

8 In the first part of the book I also expanded the section "Psychological Remarks on the Norm of Love." In so doing, I tried to relate the phenomena of loving even more primarily to the fundamental structure of the essence of human existence as it has been to us revealed to us by Martin Heidegger.[2]

32 But the nature and meaning of love can be grasped even more deeply on the basis of Martin Heidegger's fundamental ontology. On the whole, says Martin Heidegger, to be human is an ek-sisting in the literal sense of the [Latin] word *ek-sistere*. It is an original being outside itself, always out there, at or toward things and fellow human beings. Just as originally is this being-in-the-world of human beings always a being that is attuned. A first opening up and understanding of things, fellow human beings and oneself is grounded in its attunement to the world. For this attunement determines the spatiality and temporality of the world, just as does the variety and tone of all of a human being's world relations.[3]

---

1 Den abstrakten Charakter der psychoanalytischen Theorie durchschauend, glaubten die sogenannten anthropologischen' Psychopathologen, die ihre Impulse hauptsächlich von Jaspers, E. Minkowski und Heidegger empfangen hatte...

2 Ich erweiterte ferner im ersten Teil des Buches den Abschnitt über die 'Psychologischen zur Norm der Liebe.' Ich versuchte dabei, die Phänomene des Liebens noch ursprünglicher auf die fundamentalen Wesensstruktur des menschlichen Daseins zu beziehen, so wie sie uns Martin Heidegger aufgezeigt hat.

3 Noch tiefer kann das Wesen und die Bedeutung der Liebe aber auf Grund der Fundamentalontologie Martin Heideggers erfaßt werden. Mensch-sein im Ganzen, sagt Martin Heidegger, ist ein Existieren im wörtlichsten Sinne des Wortes ek-sistere. Es ist ein ursprüngliches Außer-sich-, ein Schon-immerdraußen-bei- oder zu-den-Dingen-und-Mitmenschen-Sein. Dieses In-der-Welt-sein des Menschen ist ebenso ursprünglich stets ein je gestimmtes Sein. In seiner Gestimmtheit gründet ein primäres Erschließen und Verstehen

Appendix IV

35 While, in fact, in the separateness of all possible differently determined modes of being-in-the-world men are able to see only worldly finitude and nullity,[1] as a man in loving experiences the overcoming of all strictures and anxiety, all senselessness, separateness, and nullity.[2]

40 In order to differentiate our approach from both the views of classic psychoanalysis as well as from the terminology of the previous 'anthropological' field of research, we prefer the Heideggerian term analytics of existence.[3]

---

   der Dinge der Welt, der Mitmenschen und seiner selbst. Denn diese Gestimmtheit bestimmt je und je die Räumlichkeit und Zeitlichkeit der Welt, wie die Auswahl und die Tönung aller Weltbezüge eines Menschen.

1 Note 11: "M. Heidegger [SZ 258] speaks with justification about this non-loving form of man's existing, of the "utterly unattainable possibility of death specific to it, unattested, certain and unsurpassable". Incidentally, Heidegger also unexpectedly understands that Freud's much contested conception of the death instinct can be nothing other than a drive theoretical reduction of this 'world-intentional' form of existing, of this particular constitution of existence and worldly scheme of things. But since the narrowness of the worldly finite form of existence is incommensurable with the fullness of love, it goes without saying that given the psychoanalytic abstractions of these two modes of being and their two worlds, the death instinct and the erotic instinct are not at the same level."—"M. Heidegger [SZ 258] sagt von dieser nichtliebenden Existenzform des Menschen mit Recht, es sei deren 'eigenste, unbezügliche, gewisse, und überholbare Möglichkeit der Tod.' Damit läßt übrigens Heidegger auch unversehens verstehen, daß Freuds vielumstrittene Konzeption des Todestriebes nichts anders sein kann, als die triebtheoretische Reduktion dieser 'weltlich-intentionalen' Exiztenzform, dieser besonderen Daseinsverfassung und ihres Weltenwurfes. Da aber die Enge der weltlich-endlich Existenzform mit der Fülle der Liebe inkommensurabel ist, versteht sich von selbst daß auch die psychoanalytischen Abstraktionen dieser beiden Seinsmodi und ihrer beiden Welten: Todestrieb und Erostrieb, nicht auf gleiche Ebene zu bringen sind." The passage from *Sein und Zeit* is not quoted exactly. Boss combines two formulations on the relation of existence to death found on the same page, but the sense is preserved.

2 Während faktisch die Menschen in der Vereinzelung aller möglichen andersartig gestimmten Weisen des In-der-Welt-seins nur die weltliche Endlichket und Nichtigkeit zu sehen vermögen, erlebt der Mensch als Liebender die Überwindung aller Enge und Angst, aller Sinnlosigkeit, Vereinzelung und Nichtigkeit.

3 Um dabei unsere Betrachtungsweise sowohl von den Anschauungen der klassischen psychoanalytischen Theorie wie von der bisherigen 'anthropologischen' Forschungsrichtung auch terminologisch zu unterscheiden, ziehen wir für sie den Heideggerschen Namen 'Daseinsanalytik' vor.

Appendix IV

46 Moreover, the existential-analytical way of looking at things means that anxiety is a entirely primary 'basic condition' of existence in general (Heidegger).[1]

48 Anxiety, however, is the characteristic basic condition (Heidegger) of isolated existence thrown back on itself. It is as such the most singular anthropological contrast to love and therefore also radically counteracts every expression of the fullness, breadth, depth, warmth, and eternity of the capacity for loving being-in-the-world.[2]

127 [= SG1 123]

---

1 Der daseinsanalytischen Betrachtungsweise bedeutet vielmehr die Angst eine ganz primäre 'Grundbefindlichkeit' des Daseins überhaupt (Heidegger).
2 Angst aber ist die kennzeichnende Grundbefindlichkeit (Heidegger) des auf sich selbst zurückgeworfenen, isolierten Daseins. Als solches ist sie der eigenste anthropologische Gegensatz der Liebe und stellt sich darum auch jedem Austragen der Fülle, Weite, Tiefe, Heimatlichkeit und Ewigkeit des liebend In-der-Welt-sein-könnens radikal entgegen.

Appendix V: "Nachwort" to the 3rd Edition of *Indienfahrt eines Psychiaters* (1976)

Das vorliegende Buch Indienfahrt eines Psychiaters war erstmals im Jahr 1959 im Verlag Günther Neske, Pfullingen, erschienen. 1966 wurde es ein zweites Mal, allerdings in gekürzten Form als Taschenbuch vom Herder-Verlag herausgegeben. Wenn nun der Autor und mehrere Verleger heute, zwei volle Jahrzehnte, nachdem es verfaßt worden war, miteinander übereinkommen, die Schrift noch einmal in einer dritten Auflage, doch wieder in ungekürzter und unveränderten Originalgestalt zu publizieren, müssen sie von zwei Dingen überzeugt sein. Sie hatten sich erstens darüber zu vergewissern, daß in der Zwischenzeit keine inhaltlichen Mißverständnisse zum Vorschein kamen, die in der ersten Auflage enthalten und zu korrigieren gewesen wären. Zweitens müssen sie der Auffassung sein, daß das Buch auch gegenwärtig noch nichts von seiner Aktualität eingebüßt hat.

Daß beides zutrifft, darf durch die folgenden Sachverhalte als erwiesen betrachtet werden:

Der Autor hielt sich zwar nach 1958 kein weiteres Mal leibhaftig in Indien auf. Er blieb jedoch bis heute in ununterbrochenem Kontakt mit seinen indischen Lehrern und Freunden; insbesondere mit dem im vorstehenden Text ausführlich zitierten Mahamahopadhyaya und bis zu dessen Tode vor wenigen Jahren mit demjenigen indischer Menschen, den man seinen eigentlichen "Guru" nennen könnte. Viel

Appendix V

an Bestätigung der Richtigkeit des Buchtextes erfuhr der Autor die ganze Zeit über auch von der Schweizer Psychiaterin Dr. Erna Hoch, die schon vor 18 Jahren auf sein Betreiben hin die Leitung einer psychiatrischen Klinik in Nordindien übernahm und seither ständig in Indien wirkt. Sie ist heute in ihrer beruflichen Laufbahn zum Professor für Psychiatrie an der Universität Shrinagar in Kashmir und zum Direktor der dortigen Univeraitätsklinik aufgerückt. Vor allem aber folgte sie im Bereiche des Studiums der indischen Philosophien und der hinduistischen Meditation Spuren des Autors und hielt ihn auch über ihre diesbezüglichen Erfahrungen dauernd auf dem laufenden; brieflich sowohl auch anläßlich ihrer gelegentlichen Besuche in der Schweiz.

Des weiteren führte der Autor selbst die ihm durch seine indischen Lehrer vermittelten meditativen Übungen Tag für Tag den damals empfangenen Weisungen gemäß ununterbrochen durch. Auch nach dieser Art von Erfahrung fühlt er sich zu keinen Änderungen oder Eränzungen des ursprünglichen Buchtextes veranlaßt.

Schließlich war es dem Autor vergönnt, im vergangenen Herbst für beachtliche Zeit nach Japan eingeladen zu werden, weil sich zahlreiche medizinische, philosophische und theologische Fakultäten verschiedener Universität Japans in hohem Maße für seine Daseinsanalytisches Schules interessierten. Dabei kam der Autor mit den anerkanntesten Meistern des Zen-Buddhismus Japans in nahe Berühung. Er hatte sogar das Glück, im Kreise zen-buddhistischer Mönche ausgiebig an deren meditativen Zazen-Veranstaltungen teilzunehmen. Gerade der Vergleich seiner indischen Erfahrungen mit den zen-buddhistischen Praktiken und Lehren und die dadurch möglich gewordene Abhebung jener von diesen bestätigten dem Autor aufs neue, wie sachgerecht die in diesem Buch erwähnten indischen Gegebenheiten beschrieben sind.

Nur einen einzigen Nachtrag hält der Autor an dieser Stelle und zur gegenwärtigen Zeit für angebracht und fruchtbringen bisherigen Auflagen der indienfahrt eines Psychiaters der Autor gerade die für ihn selbst überraschendste und ihn am tiefsten erschütternde Erfahrung, die ihn in Indien erwartet hatte, mit keinem Wort. Diese seine größte Überraschung darin bestanden, daß er aus dem Munde seiner indischen Gesprächspartner eine große Zahl von Sätzen zu hören bekam, die Wort für Wort dem daseinsanalytischen Werk Sein und Zeit von Martin Heidegger entnommen zu sein schienen. Dabei wüßte der Autor genau, daß weder Heidegger je etwas von den indischen Einrichten noch die indischen Weisen auch nur das Geringste von Heidegger vernommen hatten. Der Autor unterließ bis anhin jeden Hinweis darauf, weil er befürchtete, durch die Einfügung dieser Erfahrung den Verlauf der Schilderung indischer Gegebenheiten und Denkweisen, auf die es ihm allein ankam, in allzu störender Weise zu zerstückeln.

Anlaß dazu, dieses Versäumnis heute gutzumachen, gibt dem Autor eine inzwischen von seiten eines Kritikers öffentlich laut gewordene entscheidende Frage. Diese verwies ihn zunächst auf dessen Feststellung im Vorwort seiner Indienfahrt eines Psychiaters, des Inhaltes, daß er bei der seinem Aufenthalt in Indien vorangegangenen Lektüre der gesamten ihm zugänglichen Literatur über die indische Weisheit, selbst der von indischer Gelehrten verfaßten Bücher, den Verdacht nicht los wurde, in diesem Schrifttum würden durchgängig die altindischen Einsichten in die Grundverfassung des Menschen, in das Wesen seiner Welt und in die Natur des Verhältnisses beider zueinander dadurch verfälscht, daß sie gewaltsam in die westlichen platonistischen und neukantianischen Vorstellungsmodell gepreßt werden. Aber—so fuhr dann die kritische Frage fort—hat sich der Autor der Indienfahrt vor dem Anhören der indischen Weisen wohl die westliche metaphysische Brille des Platonismus und des Neukantianismus abgelegt, doch nur, um anstelle ihrer sich sogleich die ebenso westliche der Fundamental-Ontologie Martin Heideggers aufzusetzen?

Was den Autor an dieser Frage am meisten erstaunte, war weniger dies, daß sie überhaupt gestellt wurde, als vielmehr der Umstand, daß sie seines Wissens nur einmal öffentlich laut wurde. Daß nämlich in der Tat große Gefahr bestand, der Autor könnte sich in Indien in einem daseinsanalytischen Sinne ver-hören, war diesem von vornherein nur allzu bewußt; hatten ihn doch die neuen Entdeckungen Heideggers erst kurz zuvor entscheidend beeindruckt. Gerade im vollen Wissen um diese Gefahr hatte sich der Autor entsprechend gegen sie zu wappnen vermocht. Als bester Beweis für seine Unvoreingenommenheit in dieser Hinsicht mag gelten, daß der Autor auch alsogleich des

Appendix V

fundamental Unterschiedes zwischen der hinduistischen und der daseinsanalytischen Menschenkunde inne wurde. Des Westlers Heidegger tiefste Einsicht war in das, was ist, lautet: der Mensch besteht seiner Grundverfassung nach aus einem weltweit ausgespannten Vernehmenkönnen des ihm Begegnenden. Als vernehmende Erschlossenheit dieser Art wird der Mensch als jene Erscheinungsstätte in Anspruch genommen, ohne die es überhaupt nichts geben könnte. Alles nämlich, was ist und zu sein hat, bedarf eines solchen Heiligkeitibereiches, um irgendwo hinein an-wesen, in seiner Bedeutungsfülle "aufgehe", zu seinem Vorschein und damit zu seinem Sein kommen zu können.

Vom indischen Mahamahopadyaya—und nicht nur von ihm—dagegen hörte der Autor von der im vorliegenden Buchtext ausführlich erwähnten, ganz anders gearteten Erfahrung. Ihr gemäß gibt es sehr wohl einzig "Brahman", das "große Aufgehens", "Lichtung", "Gelichtetheit", "Bewußtheit" auch *ohne* Menschenwesen.

Als der Autor diesen eminenten Widerspruch, der hier zwischen den indischen Weisen und dem Westler Martin Heidegger nach seiner Rückkehr aus Indien vortrug, erwiderte dieser nach langem, nachdenklichem Schweigen: das, was er soeben vom Autor vermittelt bekommen habe, sei für Heidegger einfach nicht unmittelbar erfahrbar und könne deshalb auch für ihn nicht als Wahrheit gelten. Dies äußerte Heidegger mit genau ebenso großer Bestimmtheit, mit der dem Autor zuvor die indische Weisen ihr Wissen um menschen-unabhängiges Brahman als unmittelbarste und gewisseste meditative Erfahrung dargestellt hatten.

Entfernen sich in diesem zentralen Punkte die Einsichten indischer Weisen unüberbrückbar weit von denen der Heideggerschen Fundamental-Ontologie, rückt andererseits das vom Autor in Indien Gehörte über eine Gelichtetheit, ein Brahman, das es auch unabhängig vom Menschen, ja unabhängig von einem Gott, von Göttern oder einer Gottheit, ohne jegliches gegenüberliegendes Seiendes überhaupt gebe, in um so größere Nähe zu jener Sicht, in die sich die ursprüngliche hinduistische Erfahrung auf ihrem Weg nach Osten im Zen-Buddhismus des südlichen Japans gewandelt hat.

Appendix A: Chart Comparing the Editions

GA1 (89) Chapter Headings and Related Protocols	ZS2 Chapter Headings	[pp.]	TR3 [pp.]
[Seminar, Burghölzli September 8, 1959]	*	3-4	3-4
[Seminar, Burghölzli November, 1959]	I. Seminar	7-10]	*
[Seminar, Burghölzli February 3, 1960]	II. Seminar	21-44]	*
[Medard Boss] Conversations with Martin Heidegger in Sicily	III. Gespräche = **P I** → 637-666		
April 24 – May 6, 1963[4]	April 24 – May 4, 1963	197-226	153-181
	May 5, 1963	227	181-182
Seminar, Zollikon	IV. Seminar 89-110 Seminar 2	5-9	4-8
January 24 and 28, 1964	January 24, 1964 89-96		
	January 28, 1964 99-110		

1   The seminars [*Seminare*] are numbered I-XIII in *GA*. The second part consists of ten sets of minutes [*Protokollen*] numbered I-X. A separate part comprised of excerpts from Heidegger's letters to Boss as found in Boss's edition are not included in *GA*.
2   The *Zollikon Seminars. Protocols—Conversations—Letters* [TR] follows ZS. Any variances noted in the discussion.
3   The seminars are not numbered in *ZS*, but I have assigned them 1-11, as they are found in his edition. Likewise the conversations are not numbered, but only dated. Excerpts from Heidegger's letters to Boss are not included in *GA*.
4   Trawny refers to these conversations in *GA* § III (65-84//) but also reproduces Boss's minutes as *Protokoll* I (637-666/197-227/153-181). Boss collects the conversations in Sicily (April 24-May 4) and assigns a separate heading to notes on their flight from Rome to Zürich. Trawny includes the notes from onboard in the *Protokoll* (666/227/181-182)

GA1 (89) Chapter Headings and Related Protocols		ZS2 Chapter Headings	[pp.]	TR3 [pp.]
Seminars, Zollikon	V. Seminar 115-137	= P II → 661-690 Seminar 3	10-29	8-24
July 6 and 9, 1964	July 6, 1965	669-681	10-20	8-17
	July 9, 1965	681-690	21-29	17-24
Seminars, Zollikon	VI. Seminar 143-173	= P III → 693-708 Seminar 4	30-44	24-35
November 2 and 5, 1964	November 2, 1964	693-704	30-34	24-29
	November 5, 1964	704-708	34-44	29-35
Seminars, Zollikon	VII. Seminar 179-229	= P IV → 711-738 Seminar 5	45-52	36-56
January 18 and 21, 1965	January 18, 1965	711-722	45-66	36-44
	January 21, 1965	722-738	56-72	44-56
Seminars, Zollikon	VIII. Seminar 235-377	= P V → 741-764 Seminar 6	73-96	56-75
March 10 and 12, 1965	March 10, 1965	741-753	73-86	56-67
	March 12, 1965	754-764	86-96	67-75
Seminars, Zollikon	IX. Seminar 383-466	= P VI → 767-789 Seminar 7	97-120	75-92
May 11 and 14, 1965	May 11, 1965	767-781	97-111	75-85
	May 14, 1965	781-789	111-120	85-92

GA1 (89) Chapter Headings and Related Protocols	ZS2 Chapter Headings	[pp.]	TR3 [pp.]
Seminars, Zollikon	X. Seminar 471-557 = **PVII** → 793-817 Seminar 8	121-146	92-112
July 6 and 8, 1965	July 6, 1965 793-803	121-131	92-101
	July 8, 1965 803-817	131-146	101-112
Seminars, Zollikon	XI. Seminar 563-577 = **PVIII** → 821-847 Seminar 9	147-173	112-132
November 13 and 16, 1965[1]	November 23, 1965 821-836	147-162	112-124
	November 26, 1965 836-847	162-173	124-132
Seminars, Zollikon	XII. Seminar 583-616 = **PIX** → 851-864 Seminar 10	174-187	132-143
1 and 3 March, 1966	March 1, 1966 851-860	174-183	132-140
	March 3, 1966 860-864	183-187	140-143
Seminars, Zollikon	XIII. Seminar 621-631 = **PX** → 867-870 Seminar 11	188-191	144-147
March 18 and 21, 1969	March 18, 1969 867-868	188-189	144-145
	March 21, 1969 868-870	190-191	145-147

---

1 In the table of contents, Trawny gives the dates November 13 and 16, 1965. In *Protokoll* VIII, the minutes of the seminar (pp. 821-827) and in ZS (pp. 147-173) the dates given are November 23 and 26 1965.

Appendix B: Tables of Contents of the Three Editions

Zollikoner Seminare (GA 89, 2018) [GA]

[Seminare]

I. Zürcher Seminar November 1959

    A.   Zürcher Seminar November 1959

1. Einverständnis und Zugeständnis
2. "Sokratisch"
3. Ein einigermaßen Geordnetes Gespräch
4. Einverständnis
5. Einverständnis
6. Thesen aus Wissenschaft und Besinnung, 66
7. Verschiedene Sprachen—
8. Das Vor-läufige—
9. I.[nterpretation]
10. Versuch eines Gespräches—"mißglückt"
11. Sprache
12. Zürich
13. [Aristoteles, de anima]

    B.   Aristoteles de anima B. 1, 412A

1. Die aristotelische Bestimmung der ψυχή
2. De anima, B. 1, 412 a 3 sqq.

Appendix B

II. Burghölzli Seminar 3. Februar 1960

[A. 3. Februar 1960]

1. 3. Februar 1960
2. Gang
3. "Seinsverständnis"
   (Vorläufige Titel gebraucht in "Sein und Zeit")
4. Seinsverständnis und Sprache—Sage—Mensch und Tier
5. Mitsein
6. Mit-sein
7. Lichtenberg
8. Mit-sein
9. Burghölzli-Seminar
10. Zum Mit-sein
11. Das psychische System

[B. Aufzeichnungen zum Burghölzli-Seminar]

1. [Zur Daseinsanalyse]
2. [Das Auto]
3. Condrau—
4. [Fundamentalontologie und Psychologie]
5. [Sprache]
6. [Seminarnotiz]
7. Geschichtlichkeit des Seinsversändnisses
8. [Sinn eines psychischen Vorgangs]
9. ["Meditation"]
10. Bewußt und unbewußt—
11. Der Hinweis auf das Seinsverständnis—
12. Die Wirklichkeit—
13. [Wissenschaft und Mensch]
14. Burghölzli
15. [Burghölzli]

C. Subjektivität, Bewußstsein und Da-sein

1. Die Klärung [der] artzlichen Praxis
2. Besinnung auf das Bewußtsein

3. Die Fragen
4. [Die Fragen]
5. Edmund Husserl, Logische Untersuchungen V
6. [Da-sein und Mit-sein]
7. Dasein
8. Die erste Behauptung der Psychologie | Das Unbewußte
9. Methodische Prinzipien
10. Methodische Prinzipien
11. Freuds Rückgang
12. Die Annahme des Unbewußten
13. [Bewußtsein und Da-sein]
14. [Bewußtsein]
15. [Das Unbewußte und das Bewußte]
16. Un-bewußt
17. Das Unbewußte
18. Das Un-bewußte
19. [Das Bewußte und das Unbewußte]
20. [Das Bewußte und das Unbewußte]
21. [Sein und Zeit]
22. Fehlleistungen
23. Husserl
24. [Vergegenwärtigung]
25. Vor-stellung
26. "Die latente Erinnerung"—482!
27. Erinnerung
28. [Seminarnotiz]
29. Teilnehmer am Zollikoner Seminar (5. Februar 1960)

III. Gespräche mit Medard Boss in Sizilien vom 23. April bis 4. Mai 1963

1. [Erinnerung und Bild]
2. [Notizen zum Gespräch mit Boss]
3. Be-wußt-sein | Da-sein |
4. [Bedingung und Befugnis]
5. [Notizen zum Gespräch mit Boss]
6. Dasein—

Appendix B

7. Demeter-Hymnos
8. Verhalten—Aufenthalt—Wohnen | Welt--Ereignis
9. [Notizen zum Gespräch mit Boss]
10. [Notizen zum Gespräch mit Boss—Vergessen und Behalten]
11. Was ist ein Phänomen?
12. [Lichtung und Dasein]
13. Sein und Zeit
14. Ich—Selbst
15. [Die Erde ohne Menschen?]
16. [Die Erde ohne Menschen?]
17. [Die Erde ohne Menschen?]

IV. Phänomenologisches Seminar bei Medard Boss am 24. und 28. Januar 1964 im Anhalt an meine Schrift "Kants These über das Sein"[1]

   A. Seminar-Abend 24. Januar 1964. Gang

1. [Was ist hier vorhaben...]
2. [Lichtung und mathematische Natur]
3. ὑπόθεσις
4. [Lichtung und Sprache]
5. Annahmen
6. Das Unweisbare
7. Frage
8. "Versprechen" und Sprechen

   B. Seminar-Abend 28. Januar 1964. Gang

1. Einleitung des zweiten Abends (28. Januar)
2. [Zuletzt gelangte unser Gespräch...]
3. "Der Tisch"
4. Sprache und Metapher
5. "Verstehen"
6. ["Sinn" bei Freud]

---

1 *ZS* 5-29.

Appendix B

[V. Zum Seminar vom 6. und 9. Juli 1964]

    A.   Kausalität und Motivation Fundierung

1. Motiv—Motivation
2. Kausalität und "Satz" vom Grund
3. Grund und Gründe | Ursachen
4. [Zwang]
5. | Kausalität |

    B.   Grund—Beweis—Ausweisung "als"

1. [Gründen und Weisen]
2. Verbindlichkeit der Argumente
3. ἦ—qua—als

    [C.   Grund und Kausalität]

1. [Grund und Kausalität]
2. "Platz"
3. frei—leer
4. αἴτιον
5. Fundierung

    [D.   9. Juli 1964]

9. Juli 1964

[VI. Seminar vom 2. und 5. November 1964 in Zollikon]

    A.   Das Wesen der neuzeitlischen Naturwissenschaften und die Besinnung auf die Phänomene (2. November 1964)

1. Sokrates (469-399)
2. 2. November 1964
3. Was heißt in der neuzeitlichen Naturwissenschaft—Natur?
4. [Natur bei Kant]
5. [Kant: über Gesetz und Regel]
6. [Natur]

Appendix B

    B.   Physik

1. Die Besinnung auf "die Wissenschaft"
2. "Die Sprache der Physik". Vgl. Friedrich von Weizsäcker
3. [Physik]
4. Kreis
5. Kausalität
6. Die Einheit der Physik. Von Weizsäcker, Hütte, 19. September 1965
7. [Physik, Nietzsche]

    C.   Natur und "Kausalität"

1. Analogie der Erfahrung
2. Die naturwissenschaftliche Orientierung der neuzeitlichen Wissenschaft
3. II. Analogie
4. Psychiatrie—Psychotherapie

    D.   Das Nächstliegende

1. Das Nächstliegende
2. Begriff des "Phänomen" betrifft das "Ontologie"
3. Das Nächstliegende
4. Die Frage nach dem Einfachen—Nächstliegenden
5. Das Nächstliegende
6. Die Frage nach dem "Nächstliegende"
7. [Das Nächstliegende]
8. Ein Vorgang—eine Begebenheit
9. [Kausalität und Freiheit]

[VII. Seminar vom 18. und 21. Januar 1965 in Zollikon]

    A.   Die Frage nach der Zeit

1. Zu Platon, Timaios 37d3-38a3
2. Zeit—Chronologie
3. Jetzt sagen—
4. "Zeit her"
5. Die leitenden Horizonte in der überlieferten Vorstellung von der Zeit

Appendix B

6. "Zeit haben" und Langeweile—"Lange Zeit"
7. Wir haben keine Zeit
8. "Die Zeit haben"
9. Zeit
10. Zeit—
11. Das "in der Zeit"
12. "Zeit" und "Welt"
13. Boss
14. Langeweile—Boss-Seminar
15. "Zeit"—Boss Seminar
16. Boss-Seminar

    B. | Die Wanduhr | 21. Januar 1965]

Franz Fischer, Raum-Zeit-Struktur und Denkstörung in der Schizophrenie

    C. Boss-Seminar Januar 1965 [Zeit]

1. [Zeit]
2. [Zeit]
3. Etymologishces
4. Datum
5. Datum
6. Datum—
7. Datierung und Zeit
8. Die Uhr—Zeitmessung
9. Zeit und Zeitbewußtsein—Zeitsinn

[10. Die Fragestellung ...]

11. Zu Sein und Zeit, 498 ob [539]—Zeit und Lichtung
12. "Zeit"—
13. "Die Zeit vergeht"
14. Die Frage nach dem Eigentümlichen der Zeit

    D. Langeweile und Zeit. Vgl. WS 1929-30

1. Pascal, Pensée—Zeit und Langeweile
2. "Der Zeitvertrieb"
3. Langeweile

4. [Langeweile]
5. [Langeweile]
6. [Langeweile]
7. [Langeweile]
8. Langeweile

[VIII. Seminar vom 10. und 12. März 1965 in Zollikon]

    A.   T[emporalität]. Boss-Seminar, 10. März

[1. Es gilt ...]
2. Zeit
3. Zeit. Hegel
4. 10. März 1965

    B.   Seminar 12. März
          Zur Interpretation der Vergegenwärtigung

1. Vergegenwärtigung
2. 12. Marz 1965

    A.   März-Seminar

1. [Zeit]
2. Übersicht der bisherigen Sicht auf die Zeitphänomene
3. Zeitproblem in diesem Seminar
4. Märzseminar. Gang
5. Märzseminar. "Wanduhr"
6. Für das Märzseminar—
7. [Anschauung und Beobachtung]
8. Die Zeit selbst—ihr Eigentümliches
9. Zeit und die Zeit als solche

    [B.   Über die Zeit 1]

1. Die Charaktere der gewahrten „Zeit"
2. [Zeit]
3. Gegend—
4. [Zeit]
5. Die vor-gestellte Zeit und das Her-vor-bringen von Zeit—

Appendix B

6. Zeit
7. Zeit
8. [Zeit]
9. "In" der Zeit sein
10. [Zeit]
11. "In der Zeit". Vgl. Kant, Dissertation
12. Das "in"
13. Präposition "in"
14. ["In der Zeit"]
15. ["In der Zeit"]
16. [Zeit und Uhr]
17. Über die Atomuhr
18. "Das Jetzt-sagen" und das Zeitigen—
19. [Zeit]
20. [Zeit]
21. Zeit
22. [Zeit]
23. [Zeit]
24. Die biologische Uhr. Bünning, Portmann
25. "Technik"
26. Merke: !
27. Platon, Timaios, 37 sqq.
28. [Zeit]
29. [Zeit]
30. Die Zeitigung des Auf-Ent-Haltes
    Die gebrauchte Wahrnis der zeitenden Zeit (Lichtung)
31. Die Frage nach der Zeit als Zeit
32. Die Bezüge zur "Zeit" ‖ Die "Zeit" als Eignis
33. [Zeit]
34. Das Vordrängen der Vorstellung
35. Die Frage nach der Zeit
36. Das Zeitende der Lichtung
37. Das Nacheinander. Frage
38. Gegenwart—Gewesenheit—Zukunft (die "Zeiten" der Zeit)
39. [Zeit]
40. "Die Zeit vergeht"
41. Das "Zeit-haben" und das "Vergehen der Zeit"

Appendix B

42. "Zeit"—der zeitende. Das Geschichtliche der Zeit-erfauhrung
43. Das Zeitigne der Zeit
44. [Nahnis]
45. [Zeit]
46. [Zeit]
47. Zeit—
48. Zeit
49. Zeit—Seele—Mensch
50. [Zeit]
51. Die Zeit selbst
52. Das Jetzt im bloßen Nacheinander [reine Zeit]
53. Das Jetzt sagen—
54. Bergson
55. Zeit—als solche
56. Vorfinden der "Zeit"
57. Zeit
58. "Zeit"
59. [Zeit]
60. [Seminar in Januar 1965]
61. Das "Jetzt-Hier"
62. [Zeit]
63. [Zeit]
64. Der unmittelbare, gewohnte, aber gleichwohl nicht der tragende Bezug zur Zeit—die Uhr
65. Anfangs- und Endlosigkeit der Zeit
66. [Zeit]
67. [Zeit]
68. Die Uhr—
69. [Fachliteratur]

[C. Über die Zeit 2]

1 Hegel über die Zeit

1. Hegels Bestimmung der Zeit
2. Hegel, "Zeit" und "Ich"
3. [Hegel über die Zeit]
4. Heidegger und Hegel über die Zeit—

5. | Vermittlung | [Das Vermittelte?]
6. Das spekulative Denken
7. Hegel
8. Zeit
9. Endlichkeit und Zeit
10. Hegel
11. Hegel—"Zeit"
12. Zu Hegel: Geist und Zeit und Geschichte | vgl. dazu Sein und Zeit, § 82
13. Hegel. Zeit und Ton (Musik)

2 "Zeit". "Das Jahr" → Hegel—Kant—Lotze—Augustinus—China

1. Kant
2. Kant, Zeit
3. Zeit und Vergegenwärtigung
4. Adolf Portmann, Die Zeit im Leben der Organismen. Eranos-Jahrbuch XX, 1951, S. 454
5. Das große und das kleine Jahr
6. Baader, Vermittelung
7. Ruhe und Bewegung. Bewegung ruht in der Ruhe. → Ruhe und Zeit.
8. Franz von Baader
9. Lotze, Zeit. Der Schein eines Erscheinen.
10. Zeit und Vorstellen
11. Lotze, Zeit
12. Augustinus, tempus
13. [Augustinus, memoria]
14. Physik
15. Raum und Zeit in der Physik
16. Physik
17. Die Wandlung als das Unwandelbare

[D. Über die Zeit 3]

1. Die Frage nach der Zeit
2. [Der Anschein der Zeit]
3. Uhr und Zeitangabe

Appendix B

4. [Vergegenständlichte Zeit]
5. "Jetzt" und "Zeit"
6. "Dasein"
7. Ereignis: die wahrende Gewahrnis. Die zeitende Zeit: Die Gewährte Gewahrnis (Lichtung...)
8. "Zeit"
9. Zeit-haben und die Zeit haben
10. Uhr
11. Uhr
12. "Maß"
13. Die Uhr und Zeit-Gabe
14. Die Uhr—die gleichförmige Bewegung—"Gang"
15. "Die Zeit-haben"
16. "Uhr" und "Uhr"
17. Uhr und Zeit-haben
18. Die mythisch-Kosmische Zeit
19. Uhr
20. carpe diem
21. Die Urstiftung der "Phänomene". Zeit-Haben
22. Zeit-haben
23. "Zeit-haben"
24. "Zeit-haben"
25. [Zeiterlebnis]
26. Haben
27. [Zeit-haben]
28. Wir haben "Zeit"
29. Mensch und Zeit
30. Zahl— | zählen
31. Uhr und Technik
32. Zeitmessung
33. [Messen]
34. "Maschine"
35. "Zeitproduktion"??
36. "Die Zeit"
37. "Aufgabe" der Sanduhr
38. Die gewohnte Bedeutung von "Ereignis"

Appendix B

    E.   [Über die Zeit 4] Zeit-haben. Zeit-Messung. Die Uhr
1. Zeitangabe und Zeitgabe; Sein und Zeit, 417
2. Die Zeit geht nicht
3. 5. November [1964]
4. [Natur]
5. [Fragen]
6. [Zu Beginn der vorigen Sitzung...]
7. Das Abstrakte und die Abstraktion
8. Phänomen—Phänomenologie | Erscheinungen |
9. Uhr
10. [Zeit bei Aristoteles]
11. Zeit—Kant
12. Die Zeit als Geschenk
13. Das "Jetzt"
14. [Buch der Prediger 3,1]

[IX. Seminar vom 11. und 14. Mai 1965 in Zollikon]

    A. | Leiblichkeit und Raum |
1. [Leiblichkeit und Räumlichkeit]
2. [Das Raumhafte der Lichtung]
3. [Raum und Da-sein]
4. Verstehen—Erklären—
5. Das Problematische des Leitproblems. 14. Mai 1965
6. Phänomen
7. Zu 14. Mai. Themen
8. Zu 14. Mai. Fragen
9. 14. Mai. ["Kritik"]
10. Zu 14. Mai
11. [Grundsätze]
12. Fragen
13. Mit Leib und Seele bei—
14. Nachzuholen:
15. Leiblichkeit und Getragenheit (L)

Appendix B

B. | Psyche und Soma | Hegglin

1. "Psyche"
2. Hegglin
3. Hegglin
4. [Gefühl]

C. | Raum |

1. Raum
2. | Raum |
3. Die Räumlichkeit des Da-seins
4. Leib und Raum
5. Raum als Thema der Philosophie

B. "Leib"—"Phänomene"

1. [Mensch—Sprache—Nachricht—]
2. Nachricht (seit 17. Jahrhundert gebräuchlich)
3. "Nachricht"
4. Kybernetik—Das Prinzip der Rückkopplung
5. Da-sein—jetzt—hier
6. Leib: Leiben. Vorschlag!
7. Leib—leiben
8. "Phänomen"
9. "Leib". Vgl. zu Kybernetik
10. Leibphänomen
11. Da-sein—Leiblichkeit—Räumlichkeit
12. Mein Hiersein
13. Leib und Raum
14. Dasein und Leiblichkeit
15. In-der-Welt-sein | Leiblichkeit
16. ["Leib"]
17. "Ichheit"—"Psychisches"—Leibphänomen
18. Leibphänomen
19. "Leibphänomen"
20. Nietzsche—Der Wille zur Macht, n. 659 (1885)
21. Da-sein und Leiblichkeit

Appendix B

22. Text
23. Das Jetzt-Hier

    C.   Die Räumlichkeit des Daseins und die Leiblichkeit

1. Leiblichkeit und Räumlichkeit des Daseins
2. Durchdenke neu!
3. Thesen. Vorschlag

    D.   Raum und Leiblichkeit

1. Dasein—Raum und Leiblichkeit (vgl. Ströker, 169) nach "Sein und Zeit", 108 und 56, 137; Humanismus-Brief, 13-18
2. "Raum und Leib", Elisabeth Ströker

    E.   Ort und Raum

1. [Ort und Raum]

    F.   Getast

1. Getast und Gesicht
2. Das Getast
3. Tasten und Sehen
4. Tasten, Betasten, Berühren—

    G.   Gedächtnis und Erinnerung

1. [Zum Seminar]
2. Boss. Leib [Leib-Körper] und Dasein
3. Lichtung und Reflexion
4. Unterscheide
5. Kritik!
6. Wohin gehört "Erinnerung"?
7. Erinnerung: Ekphorieren von Engrammen.
8. Erinnerung. Das Seinerzeitige des Erlebtseins
9. Die Weise des Anwesens des Erinnerten
10. Erinnerung und Gedächtnis
11. Der Leib
12. Leib

Appendix B

13. [Leiblichkeit]
14. Leibgegebenheit und Leiben—(Leben)
15. [Weisen der Erinnerung]
16. [Henri Bergson über Erinnerung]
17. Gedächtnis und Erinnerung

    H.   Leiblichkeit—Befindlichkeit

1. Die Frage nach der Leiblichkeit
2. [Befinden]
3. [Leiblichkeit]
4. [Befinden]
5. [Leiblichkeit]
6. ["Merken" und "Spüren"]
7. [Zur Hand]
8. "Leib und Situation"

    I.   Kybernetik

1. Kybernetik
2. Kybernetik—Methode
3. Kybernetik
4. Kybernetik—Methode
5. Über das Denken Denken
2. Kybernetik

    J.   Jores

1. [Gebärde]
2. Jores
3. Jores
4. Jores

[X. Seminar vom 6. und 8. Juli 1965 in Zollikon]

    A.   Seminar am 6. Juli 1965

Seminar am 6. Juli 1965

Appendix B

B. Seminar am 8. Juli 1965

Seminar am 8. Juli 1965
[Nachtrag]

C. Zum Seminar 6. und 8. Juli 1965

1. Zum Seminar 6. und 8. Juli
2. Wahrheit. Vgl. Denken, Vorläufiges II, 38
3. [Wahrheit]
4. [Wahrheit
5. [Verhältnis und Bestimmung]
6. [Tier, Ausdruck, Leib]
7. [Wissenschaft und Phänomen]
8. Zu Seminar am 8. Juli 1965
9. [Seminarnotizen]
10. [Das Seiende]

D. Zur Methode

1. [Zur Methode]
2. Methode—μέθοδος
3. Kybernetik
4. Nietzsche über "Methode"
5. Zu Kybernetik—Methode
6. Kybernetik—
7. Kybernetik
8. Frage der Methode. Methode und Messen
9. [Methode]
10. Meßbarkeit und Methode
11. Gegenständlichkeit (Objektivität) und Meßbarkeit
12. [Meßbarkeit]
13. [Messen und Maß]
14. Meßbarkeit—
15. [Messen und Maß]
16. "Messen"
17. [Grenze]
18. "Theorie—Praxis"
19. Vorrang der Methode

Appendix B

20. "Methode"
21. [Spannen]
22. Das Meßbare
23. Meßbarkeit
24. [Messen und Zahl]
25. [Meßbarkeit]
26. [Leib und Meßbarkeit]
27. [Neuzeit und Messung]
28. [Neuzeit und Messung]
29. [Kybernetische Bestimmung des Menschen]
30. Kybernetik
31. Psychosomatik und Informationstheorie
32. [Die Definition des Menschen]

    E.   Grund (Kausalität) und Gesetz—Regel

1. Grund | Kausalität | Bedingung
2. [Bedingung und Bedingen]
3. Kausalität—Gesetz—Regel
4. Verstehen und Feststellen

    [F.   Zur Technik]

1. ["Die technische Basis"]
2. [Kommunismus und Religion]
3. Technik
4. Die Reichweite des Menschen—
5. [Sprache und Technik]
6. [Technik]
7. Ge-Stell und Steuerung
8. Maschine und Instrument
9. Weltsituation und Christentum
10. "Seiendes" und "Seinsollendes" (Wert)
11. Irrmeinung
12. Irrmeinungen! Technik
13. "Wesen der Technik"?
14. Technik und Naturwissenschaft
15. Technik. "Vorurteil"

Appendix B

16. [Technik]
17. Moderne Technik
18. [Henry Miller]
19. [Kybernetik, Wiener]
20. Das automatische Zeitalter

[G. Zu Mitsein—Mitdasein]

1. "Mit"—
2. Mit-einander—das Da-sein
3. [Zu Mit-sein]
4. Das Mitsein—Sein und Zeit, § 26—
5. In-der-Welt-sein und Person
6. Zollikoner Seminar
7. Zollikoner Seminar. Die Charakterisierung der naturwissenschaftlichen Methode
8. Zum Spruch über dem Eingang in Platons Akademie [Ontologische Differenz?]

H. In-der-Welt-sein. Ich—Du. "Gespräch" Michael Theunissen, Der Andere

1. Michael Theunissen, Der Andere
2. [Michael Theunissen, Der Andere]
3. [Da-sein]
4. Ich—Du
5. Mitdasein
6. [Michael Theunissen, Der Andere]
7. Liegt in der Auslegung des Menschseins auf das Dasein—nicht doch ein bestimmter anthropologischer Vorgriff?
8. Sein und Zeit / Methode
9. Du—als Andere
10. [Selb]
11. Das In-der-Welt-sein und die Ich-Du-Beziehung
12. Mitsein
13. In-der-Welt-sein und Ich-Du-Verhältnis
14. [Mitsein]
15. "Das dialogische Selbstwerden"

Appendix B

16. Ich-Du
17. [Mitsein und Ich-Du-Dialogik]
18. [Mitsein und Du]
19. Du—

[XI. Seminar vom 13. und 16. November 1965 in Zollikon]

    A. Daseins-Analytik—Daseinsanalyse—

1. Daseinsanalytik—Daseinsanalyse—phänomenologische Interpretation des Menschen als das Da-sein
2. "Analyse"
3. "Daseinsanalyse"
4. Die drei Vorwürfe gegen die Daseinsanalyse—
5. [Nachtrag zu 4.]
6. [Zur Daseinsanalyse]
7. "Daseinsanalytisches Denken"
8. [Zur Daseinsanalyse]
9. [Wissenschaft]
10. Begriff
11. ἀναλύσιν
12. ἀλλύω—ἀναλύσιν
13. Daseinsanalytik—Daseinsanalyse
14. Was heißt daseinsanalytisches Denken?
15. Analytik des Daseins
16. [Analytik]
17. [Analytik und Analyse]
18. [Daseinsanalytik und Daseinsanalyse]
19. Seinsfrage und Daseinsanalytik
20. Die Seinsfrage und die Analytik des Daseins
21. Da-sein—
22. [Die alltägliche Welt]
23. Die Wissenschaften und der Fachmann
24. "Daseinsanalyse"
25. Das notwendig Unzureichende der Daseinsanalytik

Appendix B

[XII. Seminar vom 1. und 3. März 1966 in Zollikon]

   A.   Stress

1. Wiederholung des Seminars vom 1. März 1966
2. Seminar 3. Marz 1966
3. Entlastung
4. Entlastung aus dem Hinblick auf die Be-anspruchung
5. Entlastung
6. [Grundstimmung der Langeweile]
7. [Wissenschaft und Denken]
8. Wissenschaft—Physik
9. Therapie
10. "Streß"— "Streß-Reiz"
11. "Streß"
12. ["Streß"]
13. "Streß"
14. Anwesenheit und Anspruch
15. Streß—Reiz (Pleonasmus)
16. Das Phänomen im Streß
17. [Reiz—Berühung—Affektion—Motiv]
18. Streß
19. Streß
20. "Streß"
21. "Streß"
22. "In-der-Welt-sein"—Wohnen
23. Reiz
24. "Ge-fühl"
25. [Plügge]
26. "Arbeitshypothese"
27. Trieb und Streben
28. Kausalität
29. [Grund und Ursache]
30. Wohnen und "Leiblichkeit"
31. Situation
32. Das Modewort "Aspekt"

Appendix B

[B. Seminar]
1. Seminar
2. Zollikoner Seminar
3. Für das nächste Seminar—Hinweise nachholen
4. [Verstehen]
5. [Mit-sein]
6. [Streß du Verstehen]
7. [Zum "Streß"]
8. [Kritik]
9. [Neuzeitliche Wissenschaft]
10. Die neuzeitliche Physik—der Vorrang der Methode—
11. "Kausalität"
12. Erklären
13. [Neuzeitliche Wissenschaft]
14. "Modell"—
15. [Psychotherapie]
16. Psychotherapie | Psychoanalyse—Daseins-analyse
17. "Analogie"
18. Freud

[XIII. Seminar vom 18. und 21. März 1969]
    A. Bewußtsein und Dasein
1. Bewußtsein und Dasein
2. Das Bewußt-sein und das Da-sein—
3. [Wissenschaft und Technik]
4. | Anerkennung | → | Tautologie |
5. Tautologie und Dialektik
6. Danken
7. Tautologie und das Eigene—
8. [Das Unverständliche]
9. [Das Sagen des Denkens und die Sache]
10. [Die Wege des Denkens]
11. [Fachliteratur]
12. [Ereignis und ...]
13. "Ereignis"
14. [Ereignis und ...]

Appendix B

15. Lichtung und Ereignis
16. Welt und Welten
17. Das Wohnen—Da-sein
18. Er-Eignis
19. "Welten"
20. Ereignis und das Ge-stelle
21. "Bewegung" und Ereignis | Lichten |
22. Hegel—Heidegger
23. [Das Da-sein]
24. [Zu Lichtung und Ort]
25. [Herbert Marcuse]
26. Kunst und "Kultur"
27. Aus "Akute psychische Begleiterscheinungen körperlicher Krankheiten" Bleuler, Willi, Bühler—1966

[Protokolle]

[I. Gespräche mit Martin Heidegger in Sizilien von 24. April bis 6. Mai 1963]
[II. Protokolle des Seminars vom 6. und 9. Juli 1964 in Zollikon]
[III. Protokolle des Seminars vom 2. und 5. November 1964 in Zollikon]
[IV. Protokolle des Seminars vom 18. und 21. Januar 1965 in Zollikon]
[V. Protokolle des Seminars vom 10. und 12. März 1965 in Zollikon]
[VI. Protokolle des Seminars vom 11. und 14. Mai 1965 in Zollikon]
[VII. Protokolle des Seminars vom 6. und 8. Juli 1965 in Zollikon]
[VIII. Protokolle des Seminars vom 23. und 26. November 1965 in Zollikon]
[IX. Protokolle des Seminars vom 1. und 3. März 1966 in Zollikon]
[X. Protokolle des Seminars vom 18. und 21. März 1969 in Zollikon]

Appendix B

Zollikoner Seminare. Protokolle–Gespräche–Briefe *(1987, 1994², 2006³) [= ZS]*

I. *Zollikoner Seminare (1959-1969)*

Seminar vom 8. September 1959 im Burghölzli[1]
Seminar vom 24. und 28. Januar [1964] im Hause Boss[2]
Seminar vom 6. und 9. Juli 1964 im Hause Boss
Seminar vom 2. und 5. November 1964 im Hause Boss
Seminar vom 18. und 21. Januar 1965 im Hause Boss
Seminar vom 10. und 12. März 1965 im Hause Boss
Seminar vom 11. und 14. Mai 1965 im Hause Boss
Seminar vom 6. und 8. Juli 1965 im Hause Boss
Seminar vom 23. und 26. November 1965 im Hause Boss
Seminar vom 1. und 3. März 1966 im Hause Boss
Seminar vom 18. und 21.März 1969

II. *Zwiegespräche mit Medard Boss*

29. November 1961, am Tage nach dem Seminar über Halluzinationen
Vom 24. April bis 5. Mai 1963, während der gemeinsamen Ferien in Taormina, Sizilien[3]
5. Mai 1963, im Flugzeug Rom—Zürich
7. September 1963, Zollikon
8. September 1963, Zollikon
29. Januar 1964, Zollikon
8. März 1965, Zollikon
12. bis 17. Mai 1965, Zollikon
8. Juli 1965, Zollikon
28. November 1965, Zollikon
29. November 1965, Zollikon
29. November 1965, Zollikon
30. November 1965, Zollikon
1965, Zollikon

---

1 Cf. GA, pp. 3-44.
2 GA, pp. 85-110 (Phänomenologisches Seminar bei Medard Boss am 24. und 28. Januar 1964 im Anhalt an meine Schrift "Kants These über das Sein")
3 GA, pp. 637-666 (*Protokoll* I).

Appendix B

6. bis 9. März 1966, Zollikon
7. Juli 1966, Zollikon
13. November 1966, Zollikon
6. Juli 1967, Zollikon
8. Juli 1967, Zollikon
22. November 1967, Zollikon
8. bis 16. März 1968, Zollikon
14. Mai 1968, Zollikon
27. September 1968, Lenzerheide
18. März 1969, Zollikon
14. Juli 1969, Zollikon
2. März 1972, Freiburg-Zähringen
3. März 1972, Freiburg-Zähringen

[[*III. Aus den Briefen an Medard Boss (1947-1971)*]]

3. August 1947
1. September 1947
15. Dezember 1947
20. März 1948
14. Juni 1948
22. Dezember 1948
2. August 1949
20. Dezember 1949
25. November 1950
15. Dezember 1950
7. März 1951
26. Januar 1952
15. März 1952
14. April 1952
2. August 1952
10. Februar 1953
30. September 1953
28. Oktober 1953
19. Dezember 1953
2. Januar 1954
11. Februar 1954
7. Juli 1954

Appendix B

10. September 1954
13. Oktober 1954
3. Januar 1955
8. Februar 1955
30. Juni 1955
17. November 1955
16. Juli 1956
29. September 1956
24. April 1957
9. Oktober 1959
9. November 1959
7. März 1960
26. März 1960
19. April 1960
10. August 1960
16. August 1960
18. Dezember 1960
1. Februar 1961
14. Februar 1961
14. März 1961
9. September 1961
15. November 1961
15. März 1962
28. Januar 1963
2. Februar 1963
3. März 1963
8. März 1963
20. März 1963
1. April 1963
11. April 1963
6. Mai 1963
1. Juni 1963
19. Juni 1963
31. August 1963
2. Oktober 1963
    Beilage zum Brief vom 2. Oktober 1963
18. Dezember 1963

Appendix B

10. Februar 1964
30. April 1964
5. Juni 1964
1. Oktober 1964
19. Oktober 1964
11. Januar 1965
4. Februar 1965
5. März 1965
3. Mai 1965
10. Juni 1965
14. Juli 1965
17. August 1965
12. September 1965
20. September 1965
26. September 1965
10. November 1965
16. Dezember 1965
18. Januar 1966
3. Februar 1966
27. März 1966
2. Juni 1966
10. Juni 1966
15. Juni 1966
15. August 1966
24. August 1966
16. Oktober 1966
4. Dezember 1966
15. Januar 1967
17. Februar 1967
5. März 1967
24. April 1967
14. August 1967
24. September 1967
1. Oktober 1967
29. Dezember 1967
10. Januar 1968
19. März 1968

Appendix B

2. April 1968
22. August 1968
7. Dezember 1968
5. Januar 1969
27. Januar 1969
7. Juli 1969
   Aus Martin Heideggers Hilfen zur Einleitung des "Grundriß-Buches"
2. August 1969
   Beilage zum 2. August 1969
20. November 1969
8. Dezember 1969
20. Februar 1970
16. August 1970
8. September 1970
21. Februar 1971
14. März 1971
2. Mai 1971

Zollikon Seminars. Protocols–Conversations–Letters *(2001)*
[= TR]

   I.   *Zollikon Seminars, 1959-1969*

   II.   *Conversations with Medard Boss, 1961-1972*

   III.   *From the Letters to Medard Boss, 1947-1971*

August 3, 1947
September 1, 1947
December 15, 1947
March 20, 1948
June 14, 1948
December 22, 1948
August 2, 1949
December 20, 1949
November 25, 1950
December 15, 1950

Appendix B

March 7, 1951
January 26, 1952
March 15, 1952
April 14, 1952
August 2, 1952
February 10, 1953
September 30, 1953
October 28, 1953
December 19, 1953
January 2, 1954
February 11, 1954
July 7, 1954
September 10, 1954
October 13, 1954
January 3, 1955
February 8, 1955
June 30, 1955
November 17, 1955
July 16, 1956
September 29, 1956
April 24, 1957
October 9, 1959[1]
November 9, 1959
March 7, 1960
March 26, 1960
April 19, 1960
August 10, 1960
August 16, 1960
December 18, 1960
February 1, 1961
February 14, 1961
March 14, 1961
September 9, 1961
November 15, 1961
March 15. 1962

---

1 *ZS* reads October 19, 1959.

Appendix B

January 28, 1963
February 2, 1963
March 3, 1963
March 8, 1963
March 20, 1963
April 1, 1963
April 11, 1963
May 6, 1963
June 1, 1963[1]
June 19, 1963
August 31, 1963
October 2, 1963
    Enclosure with the Letter of October 2, 1963, from Todtnauberg
December 18, 1963
February 10, 1964
April 30, 1964
June 5, 1964
October 1, 1964
October 19, 1964
January 11, 1965
February 4, 1965
March 5, 1965
May 3, 1965
June 10, 1965
July 14, 1965
August 17, 1965
September 12, 1965
September 20, 1965
September 26, 1965
November 10, 1965
December 16, 1965
January 18, 1966
February 3, 1966 [75]
March 27, 1966
June 2, 1966

---

1   *ZS* reads July 1, 1963.

Appendix B

June 10, 1966
June 15, 1966
August 15, 1966
August 24, 1966
October 16, 1966
December 4, 1966
January 15, 1967
February 17, 1967
March 5, 1967
April 24, 1967
August 14, 1967
September 24, 1967
October 1, 1967
December 29, 1967
January 10, 1968
March 19, 1968
April 2, 1968
August 22, 1968
December 7, 1968
January 5, 1969
January 27, 1969
July 7, 1969
   Enclosure with the Letter of July 7, 1969: With Heidegger's Assistance with the Introduction to the *Foundations* Book
August 2, 1969
   Enclosure to the Letter of August 2, 1969
November 20, 1969
December 8, 1969
February 20, 1970
August 16, 1970
September 8, 1970
February 21, 1971
March 14, 1971
May 2, 1971

Appendix C: Notes on Trawny's Manuscript Sources

[873] B 56, 6 Zürich Seminar. Burghölzli, November 1959 (20 sheets of paper) {7-16}
B 56, 6 Burghölzli, February 3, 1960 (14 sheets of paper) {21-27}
B 56,6 [Notes of the Burghölzli Seminar] (20 sheets of paper) {31-44}
B 56, 6 Subjectivity, Consciousness and There-being (March 1960) (31 sheets of paper) {47-61}
B 59, 3 Sicily. Conversations with Medard Boss, April 23 to May 4, 1963 (27 sheets of paper) with [a] record of conversations with Prof. Martin Heidegger in Taormina, Sicily, from April 24 to May 6, 1963 (18 sheets of paper) {65-84}
B 74,1 Seminar in connection with the paper "Kant's Thesis about Being" (37 sheets of paper) with minutes from July 6 and 9, 1964 (9 sheets of paper) {89-110}
B 58,8 Causality and Motivation. Foundations (23 sheets of paper) {115-131}
D 1,5 [July 9, 1964] (5 sheets of paper) {135-137}
B 32, 7 Das Essence of Contemporary Natural Science and Reflection on the Phenomenon (November 2, 1964) (10 sheets of paper) {143-150}
B 32,7 Physics (19 sheets of paper) {153-161}
B 32,7 Nature und "Causality" (5 sheets of paper) {165-166}
B 32, 7 The Nearby (12 sheets of paper) {169-173}
B 71 The Question Concerning Time I. January 18 and 21, 1965 (81 sheets of paper) {179-229}
B 32, 8 T[emporality]. Boss Seminar, March 10, 1965, and On the Inter-

Appendix C

pretation of Visualization. Seminar, March 12, 1965 (44 sheets of paper) {235-257} [VIII "A.¹"]

B 71 March Seminar (1965) (13 sheets of paper) {261-280} [VIII "B.²" and "A.³"] + On Time 1 {283-314} [VIII "[B.⁴"]

B 71 The Question Concerning Time II[2(-4)] (266 sheets of paper) {319-377}

C 2, 10 Corporeality and Space (55 sheets of paper) {383-417} [IX "B.⁵" and "C.⁶" and "B.⁷"

C2, 11a The Spatiality of Existence and Corporeality (3 sheets of paper) {420-422} ["C.⁸"]

C2, 11b Space and Corporeality (7 sheets of paper) {425-429}

C2, 11c Place and Space (1 sheet of paper) {433}

C2, 11d Touch (4 sheets of paper) {437-438}

C22, 3b Recollection and Memory (17 sheets of paper) {441-449}

B 58, 8 Corporeality and Situatedness. See *BaT* [*Being and Time*], § 28 ff. (9 sheets of paper) {453-466}

B 32, 7 Seminar of July 6 and 8, 1965 (96 sheets of paper) {471-524}

B 32, 8 [On Technology] (20 sheets of paper) {527-537}

B 58, 8 [Togetherness and Coexistence] (10 sheets of paper) {541-544}

B 58, 8 Being-in-the-world. I—Thou. "Conversation" (32 sheets of paper) {547-557}

B 58, 8 Analytics of Existence. Existential Analysis (Seminar, November 1965) (33 sheets of paper) {563-577}

B 58, 8 Seminar, March 1 and 3, 1966 (38 sheets of paper) {583-616}

C 2, 1 Consciousness and Existence (March 1969) (29 sheets of paper) {621-631}

Yellow Portfolio 15 [Minutes with handwritten notations] (74 sheets of paper)⁹ -- *Protokolle* [?] {637-870}

---

1   <A. T[emporalität]. Boss-Seminar, 10. März> {235-257}
2   <B. Seminar 12. März. Zur Interpretation der Vergegenwärtigen> {261-272}
3   <A. März-Seminar> {275-280}
4   <[B. Über die Zeit 1]> {283-314}
5   <B. | Psyche und Soma> | Hegglin {397-398}
6   <C. | Raum |> {401-403}
7   <B. "Leib"—"Phänomene"> {407-417}
8   <C. Die Räumlichkeit des Daseins und die Leiblichkeit> {421-422}
9   The [manuscript] titles are the headings given by Heidegger. Titles placed in square brackets were added by me. The upper case letters B, C and D represent

Appendix D: Notes on the Boss Edition

Zollikoner Seminare. Protokolle–Gespräche–Briefe *(1987, 1994², 2006³) [= ZS]*

I. *Zollikoner Seminare (1959-1969)*

Seminar vom 8. September 1959 im Burghölzli[1]
Seminar vom 24. und 28. Januar [1964] im Hause Boss[2]
Seminar vom 6. und 9. Juli 1964 im Hause Boss
Seminar vom 2. und 5. November 1964 im Hause Boss[3]
Seminar vom 18. und 21. Januar 1965 im Hause Boss
Seminar vom 10. und 12. März 1965 im Hause Boss
Seminar vom 11. und 14. Mai 1965 im Hause Boss
Seminar vom 6. und 8. Juli 1965 im Hause Boss

---

an outline of the manuscripts, which Hermann Heidegger in collaboration with Friedrich-Wilhelm von Herrmann produced during long years of archival work at the German literary archive in Marbach am Neckar in the form of a list of Heidegger manuscripts.

1 Cf. GA, pp. 3-44. [Note 3/337: Verbatim minutes oft he entire seminar are missing. The only thing that was recorded was the probably unique graphic representation of there-being [*Da-sein*] which was sketched by Martin Heidegger in chalk on the blackboard of the auditorium. It looked like the above. A written note by Heidegger on it follows the drawing.
2 GA, pp. 85-110 (Phänomenologisches Seminar bei Medard Boss am 24. und 28. Januar 1964 im Anhalt an meine Schrift "Kants These über das Sein")
3 [Note 30/24: The first session for November 2, 1964, is headed "Introduction to an Anecdote on Socrates."]

Appendix D

Seminar vom 23. und 26. November 1965 im Hause Boss
Seminar vom 1. und 3. März 1966 im Hause Boss
Seminar vom 18. und 21.März 1969

II. *Zwiegespräche mit Medard Boss (1961-1972)*[1]

29. November 1961, am Tage nach dem Seminar über Halluzinationen
Vom 24. April bis 5. Mai 1963, während der gemeinsamen Ferien in Taormina, Sizilien[2]
5. Mai 1963, im Flugzeug Rom—Zürich
7. September 1963, Zollikon[3]
8. September 1963, Zollikon
29. Januar 1964, Zollikon
8. März 1965, Zollikon[4]

---

1 [Note 193/149: Subtitle for Part Two's title page: Statements by Martin Heidegger taken down during his conversations with Medard Boss during his visits to Boss's home and on a holiday taken together.] [Note 197-226/153-181: Subheadings within the entry are: Galileo's and Newton's Concept of Nature (198/153), Discussion of Physiological Explanations (199/155), Addendum (201/156), On the Concept of Representation (206/161), On Perception of Other People (207/162), On Introjection (208-163), On Projection (208/193), On Transference (210/165), On the Term 'Projective Test' (211/165), On Affects (211/166), On Therapy (212/167), On Forgetting (212165), On Remembering (215/170), On Willing, Wishing, Propensity, and Urge (217/172), On the 'Psychical Functions': Ego, Id, Superego [I, It, Over Me] (220/174), On: Essence and Concept of Essence (220/175), On: Being and Existence [Sein und Dasein] (221/176). [Note (199/155) Boss concludes the section on "Galileo's and Newton's Concept of Nature" with this parenthetical comment" [Refers to Mrs. Zürcher in the Outline [Grundriß-Buch] by Medard Boss.] The complete title of the second edition is given in the footnote: *Outline of Medicine and Psychology. Approaches to a Phenomenological Physiology, Psychology, Pathology, Therapy and to an Existential Preventive Medicine* (Bern: Huber, 1974).]
2 *GA*, pp. 637-666 (*Protokoll* I). [Note 197/153: Following the dates, Boss writes: ... during their vacation taken together in Taormina.]
3 [Note 228-229/339: Refers to the place in Freud's writings where he expresses his realization that words or language belong to consciousness, but at the same time admits that children, who while they play with things but cannot yet speak, cannot be said to be without consciousness. Freud concludes his description of these facts with words of resignation, that here everything is still in the dark.]
4 [Note 236/339: Martin Heidegger's handwritten text.] [Note 238/339: Referring to text in response to the question "What is the meaning of the 'reception of *Being and Time* for psychiatry?" (238-242/191-195): Heidegger jotted on little scraps of

Appendix D

12. bis 17. Mai 1965, Zollikon[1]
8. Juli 1965, Zollikon[2]
28. November 1965, Zollikon
29. November 1965, Zollikon[3]
29. November 1965, Zollikon[4]
30. November 1965, Zollikon
1965, Zollikon
6. bis 9. März 1966, Zollikon
7. Juli 1966, Zollikon
13. November 1966, Zollikon[5]
6. Juli 1967, Zollikon
8. Juli 1967, Zollikon
22. November 1967, Zollikon
8. bis 16. März 1968, Lenzerheide[6]

---

    paper (mostly in keywords) the following critique of Binswanger's opinion about Being-in the-world and transcendence.]
1 [Note (247/198) preceding his commentary, the passage Heidegger comments is given: [What follows is Martin Heidegger's commentary on the World Health Organization's report on psychosomatic disorders as reported by [Werner] Schwidder in the *Zeitschrift für psychosomatische Medizin* (*Journal of [P]sychosomatic [M]edicine* 11(2), 1965, pp. 146 ff. The text reads:]]
2 [Note (251/202) re Heidegger's comments (251/202): Remarks on Professor Akeret's report on recollection, July 10, 1965, at the Burghölzli. Note (251/202) re Heidegger's on affect: [On Heidegger's discussions of 'affects' in his book on Nietzsche:]]
3 [Note (254/204) Boss adds to the date: Remarks on Blankenburg's critique. Note 254/339: Reference to an article by Wolfgang Blankenburg (1965). Note (257/339) Reference to article by Ludwig Binswanger (1946).]
4 [Note (258/206) Boss adds to the date: Remarks on Boss's planned lectures in Argentina in 1966.]
5 [Note (266/339) Heidegger's handwritten text. Note (266): The ZS text provides a heading for the section (266) which is missing in TR: On the role of the perspective of genetics.]
6 [Note (273/340) re Heidegger's discussion of Part Two of the manuscript of Boss's book, which Boss refers in its second, expanded edition (1975): M. Boss, *Grundriß der Medizin und der Psycholgie*. The following topic headings refer to the manuscript of this book which was in the process of being realized at that time. TR adds: "See Boss, *Existential Foundations*, p. 85 ff." This was Chapter 7, which contained sections on the spatiality and temporality of *Da-sein*, *Leiblichkeit* and much more. What matters is realizing that *Grundriß* was already in evidently well-organized manuscript form by 1968.] [Note (274/340) Boss writes: Refers to symptoms of a patient mentioned in the book Grundriß der Medizin. Here Boss

Appendix D

14. Mai 1968, Zollikon
27. September 1968, Lenzerheide[1]
18. März 1969, Zollikon
14. Juli 1969, Zollikon
2. März 1972, Freiburg-Zähringen[2]
3. März 1972, Freiburg-Zähringen

[[III. *Aus den Briefen an Medard Boss (1947-1971)*]]

3. August 1947
1. September 1947
15. Dezember 1947
20. März 1948
14. Juni 1948
22. Dezember 1948
2. August 1949
20. Dezember 1949
25. November 1950
15. Dezember 1950
7. März 1951
26. Januar 1952
15. März 1952
14. April 1952
2. August 1952
10. Februar 1953
30. September 1953
28. Oktober 1953

---

uses the original title (1971), minus "… *und Psychologie.*" TR refers to pp. 3-17 of *Existential Foundations*, Boss's initial presentation of the "test case," Regula Zürcher. TR also refers the reader to Boss's note that *first* mentions his book (199/339) with its complete German title. Reference is made to TR, pp. 3-17.]

1 [Note (279/340) Heidegger's handwritten text. Note (279/340) The headings and page numbers refer to Medard Boss's *Outline* [*Grundriß-Buch*] which was in the process of coming into being. The reader is referred to reference (273/340).]

2 [Note 288/340) The basis of the conversation is the working out of the second dream book by the editor: Medard Boss, *Er träumte mir vergangene Nacht…. Sehübungen im Bereiche des Träumens und Beispiele für die praktische Anwendung eines neuen Traumverständnisses* (Bern: Huber, 1975). Mercifully, the English translation of 1977 is not mentioned.]

Appendix D

19. Dezember 1953
2. Januar 1954
11. Februar 1954
7. Juli 1954
10. September 1954
13. Oktober 1954
3. Januar 1955
8. Februar 1955
30. Juni 1955
17. November 1955
16. Juli 1956
29. September 1956
24. April 1957
9. Oktober 1959
9. November 1959
7. März 1960
26. März 1960
19. April 1960
10. August 1960
16. August 1960
18. Dezember 1960
1. Februar 1961
14. Februar 1961
14. März 1961
9. September 1961
15. November 1961
15. März 1962
28. Januar 1963
2. Februar 1963
3. März 1963
8. März 1963
20. März 1963
1. April 1963
11. April 1963
6. Mai 1963
1. Juni 1963
19. Juni 1963

Appendix D

31. August 1963
2. Oktober 1963
   Beilage zum Brief vom 2. Oktober 1963
18. Dezember 1963
10. Februar 1964
30. April 1964
5. Juni 1964
1. Oktober 1964
19. Oktober 1964
11. Januar 1965
4. Februar 1965
5. März 1965
3. Mai 1965
10. Juni 1965
14. Juli 1965
17. August 1965
12. September 1965
20. September 1965
26. September 1965
10. November 1965
16. Dezember 1965
18. Januar 1966
3. Februar 1966
27. März 1966
2. Juni 1966
10. Juni 1966
15. Juni 1966
15. August 1966
24. August 1966
16. Oktober 1966
4. Dezember 1966
15. Januar 1967
17. Februar 1967
5. März 1967
24. April 1967
14. August 1967
24. September 1967

Appendix D

1. Oktober 1967
29. Dezember 1967
10. Januar 1968
19. März 1968
2. April 1968
22. August 1968
7. Dezember 1968
5. Januar 1969
27. Januar 1969
7. Juli 1969
   Aus Martin Heideggers Hilfen zur Einleitung des "Grundriß-Buches"
2. August 1969
   Beilage zum 2. August 1969
20. November 1969
8. Dezember 1969
20. Februar 1970
16. August 1970
8. September 1970
21. Februar 1971
14. März 1971
2. Mai 1971

An International Bibliography of the Writings of Medard Boss (1929-2003)

INTRODUCTORY NOTE

The literary output of Medard Boss (1903-1990) consists of 13 books, contributions to 34 edited volumes, 12 co-authored essays and two co-edited volumes, 86 journal articles, and his edition of Martin Heidegger's *Zollikon Seminars*. His little known introduction to Carlos Alberto Seguín's *Love and Psychotherapy. The Psychotherapeutic Eros* is essential reading on the meaning of genuine psychotherapy. Boss wrote in German and English. He was also at home in French, Italian, and Spanish and in his later years read conference papers in Portuguese. He has been translated into these and other languages, including Dutch, Japanese, Russian and Swedish. Regrettably, a great deal of his work has not yet been translated into English. Most of it that has is of poor quality.

Boss contributed to meetings held in both of the Americas, in India, and throughout Europe and the United Kingdom. His experiences as a physician, psychotherapist and philosopher are recounted in his charming memoir (1973) which I have recently translated into English for publication.

Many of his papers are devoted to psychosomatics and schizophrenia, topics that occupied Boss's attention as a physician and psychiatrist throughout his career, but the bulk of his work that is of the greatest interest now when the future of psychotherapy is uncertain is devoted to working out and articulating the unique approach to psychoanalysis that slowly evolved during his close study of the work of Martin Heidegger: *Daseinsanalyse*. This was his final preferred "American translation" of the German term as it appears in his preface to *Zollikon Seminars* (2001).

By contrast with Ludwig Binswanger's earlier appropriation of Heidegger's *Daseinsanalytik* (analytics of existence) for psychiatry, Boss's understanding of Heidegger's ontology of existence (*Da-sein*) for therapeutics merited Heidegger's approval. It followed many years of close tutorial and personal collaboration with the philosopher, culminating in the well-known series of seminars for psychiatrists, psychotherapists and others directed by Heidegger between 1959 and 1969 at Boss's office in the Zollikon district of Zürich. Although the reader will find the influence of Heidegger as early as 1947 in Boss's book on the paraphilias (then termed perversions), in 1971 it reached its maturity in his comprehensive discussion of medicine and psychology, parts of which were written by Heidegger, who examined and edited the entire work—his outline of medicine and psychology on existential principles.

This bibliography is intended to provide students of psychology, practicing psychotherapists, and psychiatrists with an overview of Boss's interests, including medicine, psychiatry, philosophy, psychology and the human sciences, and even certain social issues that concerned him. Access to some of these texts is challenging. Sadly, all but one of his books in English translation are now out of print. Apart from his pioneering *Psychoanalyse und Daseinsanalytik* [*Psychoanalysis and the Analytics of Existence*] (1957) and the *Grundriß der Medizin* [*und der Psychologie*]. *Ansätze zu einer phänomenologischen Physiologie, Psychologie, Pathologie, Therapie und zu einer daseinsgemäßen Präventiv-Medizin in der modernen Industrie-Gesellschaft* [*Outline of Medicine [and Psychology]. Approaches to a Phenomenological Physiology, Psychology, Pathology, Therapy and to an Existentially Informed Preventative Medicine*] (1971; rev. ed. with new title, 1975), two books on dreaming and dreams (1953, 1975) merit special attention. In 1979, Boss selected what he took to be his 25 most important papers from 1937 to 1978 and published them as *Von der Psychoanalyse zur Daseinsanalyse. Wege zu einem neuen Selbstverständnis* [**From Psychoanalysis to Daseinsanalysis. Paths to a New Self-Understanding**] (1979). A few years later he did this again with *Von der Spannweite der Seele. Ausgewählte Vorträge und Aufsätze aus den Anwendungsbereichen des daseinsanalytischen Menschenverständnisses* [**On the Wingspan of the Soul. Selected Lectures and Essays from Areas of Application of the Existential Analytic Understanding of Man**] (1982) which brings together 13 papers written between 1974 and 1981. Perhaps the most unique among his texts, however, is *Indienfahrts eines Psychiaters* [**A Psychiatrist's Journey to India**] (1959), which Boss claimed was his "favorite" book and prompted my article on Boss, Heidegger, Near Eastern philosophy, and psychotherapy.[1]

The following items are arranged chronologically by genre. Items **bolded** are English translations. The translator is given, if known. Apart from the papers he wrote in English, it is likely that when a translator is not given it was Boss himself who prepared it. These are marked (B).

Since Boss has not been well represented in English translation, for each entry I have offered what I think is a helpful English title of the contribution in square brackets based on my Glossary of suggested translation decisions.

The bibliography concludes with a list of awards and other forms of recognition accorded Boss in the course of his career. Finally, I have added a Chronological List of Publications using my working English titles and an Index that reflects the major themes of interest to Boss dealt with in his publications. An earlier version of the bibliography prepared by Medard Boss and revised by Marianne Boss-Linsmayer was made available to me to see to publication (see 2002/2003, below). Many errors in that manuscript have been corrected and additional publications were discovered.

At this time, I am unaware of any plans to prepare revised translations of his books, although this is much to be desired. A German collected edition of Boss's publications would be welcome.

---

1 "Medard Boss and Martin Heidegger. The Existential Analyst as 'a Western Kind of *rishi*,'" in *Review of Existential Psychology and Psychiatry* **27** (1-3), 2008, pp. 43-60.

An International Bibliography of the Writings of Medard Boss

I. BOOKS

1. *Körperliches Kranksein als Folge seelischer Gleichgewichtsstörungen* (Bern: Huber, 1940; 6th ed. 1978). [*Physical illness as a result of psychological imbalance*]

    [Swedish translation: *Själsharmoni och hälsa* (Stockholm: Natur und Kultur, 1944)]
    [Japanese translation: *Shinshin igaku nyūmon* (Tokyo: Misuzu Shobo, 1959, 1966)].

2. *Die Bedeutung der Psychologie für die menschlichen Lebens- und Arbeitsgemeinschaften* (Thalwil-Zürich: Oesch, 1943; 3rd ed. 1950). [*The significance of psychology for human relationships and community life*]

3. *Die Gestalt der Ehe und ihre Zerfallsformen. Ein Beitrag zur Psychopathologie der menschlichen Gemeinschaftsbildungen* (Bern: Huber, 1944).
    [*The shape of marriage and its forms of disintegration. A contribution to the psychopathology of the formation of human community life*]

4. *Sinn und Gehalt der sexuellen Perversionen. Ein daseinsanalytischer Beitrag zur Psychopathologie des Phänomens der Liebe* (Bern: Huber, 1947; 2nd revised and expanded ed., 1952, which contains a new "Vorwort [Preface]"; Munich: Kindler, 3rd, further revised and expanded ed., 1966, which contains a new "Vorwort [Preface] (pp. 9-13)" and an important "Nachwort [Postscript]" (pp. 174-182); 4th ed., Frankfurt: Fisher, 1984; 2017).
    [*Meaning and content of sexual perversions. A existential-analytical contribution to the psychopathology of the phenomenon of love*]

    [English translation: *Meaning and Content of Sexual Perversions. A Daseinsanalytic Approach to the Psychopathology of the Phenomenon of Love* (New York: Grune and Stratton, 1949).] (Lise Lewis Abell)
    [Japanese translation: *Seiteki tōsaku: Ren'ai no seishin byōrigaku* (Tokyo: Misuzu Shobo, 1957, 1998)]

[Italian translations: *Senso e contenuto delle perversioni sessuali* (Milan: Sugor, 1962); *Perversioni sessuali: significati e contenuti* (Milan: Vivarium, 1998)]

5. *Der Traum und seine Auslegung* (Bern: Huber, 1953; 2nd ed., Munich: Kindler, 1974).
   [The dream and its interpretation]

   [English translation: *The Analysis of Dreams* (New York: Philosophical Library, 1958).] (Arnold J. Pomerans)
   [Japanese translation: *Yume : Sono gensonzai bunseki* (Tokyo: Misuzu Shobo, 1970)].

6. *Einführung in die psychosomatische Medizin* (Bern: Huber, 1954).
   [*Introduction to psychosomatic medicine*]

   [French translation: *Introduction à la médicine psychosomatique* (Paris: Presses Universitaires, 1959)].

   An abridged version was published as *Praxis der Psychosomatik. Krankheit und Lebensschicksal* (Bern: Benteli, 1978).
   [*Practice of Psychosomatics. Illness and Personal Fate*]

7. *Psychoanalyse und Daseinsanalytik* (Bern: Huber, 1957; 2nd ed., 1980).
   [*Psychoanalysis and the analytics of existence*]

   [Dutch translation: *Psychoanalyse en daseinsanalyse* (Utrecht: Bijleveld, 1958)]
   [Spanish translation: *Psicoánalisis y analítica existential* (Madrid: Javier Morata, 1958)]
   [Japanese translation: *Seishin bunseki to gensonzai bunsekiron* (Tokyo: Misuzu Shobo, 1962)]

   [English translation: *Psychoanalysis and Daseinsanalysis* (New York: Basic Books, 1963; 2nd ed., New York: Dacapo Press, 1982)] (Ludwig B. Lefebre; Elsa Lehman and Mary Hottinger-Mackie)
   [Italian translation: *Psicoanalisi e analitica esistenziale* (Rome: Astrolabio), 1973].
   [French translation: *Psychanalyse et Analytique du Dasein* (Paris: Vrin, 2007].

8. *Indienfahrt eines Psychiaters* (Pfullingen: Neske, 1959; 2nd ed., Freiburg: Herder, 1966; 3rd ed., Bern: Huber, 1976; 4th, expanded and illustrated ed., Bern: Huber 1987; 5th ed., Bern: Huber, 2006). The final chapter, "Eastern Wisdom and Western Psychotherapy" (pp. 184-192), was reprinted in John Welwood (ed.), *The Meeting of the Ways* (New York: Schocken, 1979), pp. 183-191.
[*A psychiatrist's journey to India*]

   [English translation: *A Psychiatrist Discovers India* (London: Wolff, 1965).] (Henry A. Frey)
   [Swedish translation: *Indisk visdom och modern psykiatrie* (Stockholm: Natur och Kultur, 1967)]
   [French translation: *Un psychiatre en Inde* (Paris: Fayard, 1971)]
   [Japanese translation: *Tōyō no eichi to seiō no shinri ryōhō: seishin igakusha no indo kikō* (Tokyo: Misuzu Shobo, 1972)].

   [An important postscript was added to the third edition (pp. 261-263). The 4th edition includes "After Thirty Years. Preface to *A Psychiatrist Journeys to India* (4th Edition)" [1987], in *Review of Existential Psychology and Psychiatry* **27**(1-3), 2002-2003, pp. 33-36. Reprinted as a monograph by Keith Hoeller (ed.), *The Heidegger-Boss Relationship* (Seattle: Review of Existential Psychology and Psychiatry, 2008), pp. 33-36.]

9. *Lebensangst, Schuldgefühle und psychotherapeutische Befreiung* (Bern: Huber, 1962; 2nd ed., 1965) [LSB].
   [Fear of life, feelings of guilt, and psychotherapeutic liberation]

   [English translation: "Anxiety, Guilt and Psychotherapeutic Liberation," in *Review of Existential Psychology and Psychiatry* 2, 1962, pp. 173-195 [REPP]. Reprinted in Keith Hoeller (ed.), *Readings in Existential Psychology and Psychiatry* (Seattle: Review of Existential Psychology and Psychiatry, 1990), pp. 71-92]. (B)
   [Japanese translation: *Fuan no seishin ryoho* (Kyoto: Daigoshobo, 2000]

   Contents:
   [Vorwort: LSB 9-12 (Introduction to the 5th International Congress of Psychotherapy, August 21-26, 1961.]

Anxiety and Guilt as Basic Powers of Human Life [Angst und Schuld als Grundmächte des Menschlebens: LSB 13-17] (= REPP 173-175)
Psychological Explanations as Intellectual Short-Circuits [Die psychologischen Erklärung als gedankliche Kurzschlüsse: LSB 18-25] (= REPP 175-178]
Quest for a New Mindfulness [Versuch einer neuen Besinnung: LSB 26-28] (= REPP 178-183)
The Way into the Open [Der Weg ins Freie: LSB 39-52] (= REPP 183-189)
The New Mindfulness as Foundation of the Possibility of Therapeutic Liberation [Die neue Besinnung als Fundament psychotherapeutischer Befreiungsmöglichkeiten: LSB 53-62] (= REPP 189-195].

10. *Grundriß der Medizin. Ansätze zu einer phänomenologischen Physiologie, Psychologie, Pathologie, Therapie und zu einer daseinsgemäßen Präventiv-Medizin in der modernen Industrie-Gesellschaft* (Bern: Huber, 1971; 2nd, expanded ed., 1975; 3rd ed., 1999, with a "Preface" by Marianne Boss; new title beginning with 2nd ed.: *Grundriß der Medizin und der Psychologie. Ansätze zu einer phänomenologischen Physiologie, Psychologie, Pathologie, Therapie und zu einer daseinsgemäßen Präventiv-Medizin in der modernen Industrie-Gesellschaft*].
[*Outline of medicine and psychology. Approaches to a phenomenological physiology, psychology, pathology, therapy and to an existentially informed preventative medicine*]

[English translation: *Existential Foundations of Medicine and Psychology* (New York: Jason Aronson, 1979).] (Stephen Conway and Anne Cleaves)
[Slovak translation: *Nárys medicíny a psychológie* (Bratislava: ObNV, 1985)].

11. *"Es träumte mir vergangene Nacht...": Sehübungen im Bereiche des Träumens und Beispiele für praktische Anwendung eines neuen Traumverständnisses* (Bern: Huber, 1975; 2nd ed. 1991).
[*"It dreamt me last night...": Visual exercises in the sphere of dreaming and examples of the practical use of a new understanding of the dream*]

[Croatian translation: *Novo tumacenje snova* ... (Zagreb: Naprijed, 1985)]
[English translation: *"I dreamt last night...": A New Approach to the Revelations of Dreaming—and Its Uses in Psychotherapy* (New York: Gardner Press, 1977; 2nd ed., 1988)] (Stephen Conway)
[Portuguese translation: *Na noite passada eu sonhei...* (Sao Paulo: Ed. Summus, 1979)]
[French translation: *Il m'est venu en rêve...* (Paris: Presses Universitaires, 1989)]
[Czech translation: *Vcera v noci se mi zdálo...* (Prague: Grada, 1994; Triton, 2002)]

12. *Von der Psychoanalyse zur Daseinsanalyse. Wege zu einem neuen Selbstverständnis* (Vienna: Europaverlag, 1979).
[*From psychoanalysis to analysis of existence. Paths to a new self-understanding*]

Contents:
"Die Grundprinzipien der Schizophrenietherapie im historischen Rückblick" [1937]: pp.11-53.
"Individuelle Vorbehandlung zur kollektiven Arbeitstherapie bei schweren, chronischen Schizophrenen" [1938]: pp. 55-70.
"Über drei Kategorien vermeidbarer Mißerfolge in der ärztlichen Allgemeinpraxis" [1939]: pp. 71-93.
"Alte und neue Schocktherapien und Schocktherapeuten" [1941]: pp. 95-103.
"Die Möglichkeiten und Grenzen der Psychotherapie" [1948]: pp. 105-121.
"Vom Weg und Ziel der tiefenpsychologischen Therapie" [1948]: pp. 123-144.
"Beitrag zur daseinsanalytischen Fundierung des psychiatrischen Denkens" [1951]: pp. 145-150.
"Die Bedeutung der Daseinsanalyse für die Psychologie und die Psychiatrie" [1952]: pp. 151-160.
"Psychoanalyse eines Sadisten" [1952]: pp. 151-160.
"Die Psychotherapie des praktischen Arztes" [1959]: pp. 187-202.

"Einem Therapeuten wird sein bio-psychologischer Star gestochen" [1953/1957]—[Source given as a combination of an adaptation of "Martin Heidegger und die Ärzte" [1959, pp. 276-290] and material from the first chapter of what Boss cites as *Psychoanalysis and Daseins-Analysis* ["A Patient Who Taught the Author to See and Think Differently"], the English "translation" (1963) of the first edition of his *Psychoanalyse und Daseinsanalytik* [1957]: pp. 203-244.
"Daseinsanalytische Bemerkungen zu Freuds Vorstellung des 'Unbewußten'" [1960-61]: pp. 245-266.
"Die Bedeutung der Daseinsanalyse für die psychoanalytische Praxis" [1960-61]: pp. 267-285.
"Begegnung in der Psychotherapie" [1964]—[Source given as "Vortragsmanuskript" [1965]; but see "Begegnung in der Psychotherapie," in *Psychotherapy and Psychosomatics* 13(5), 1965, pp. 332-341]: pp. 287-294.
"Die sexuellen Perversionen in phänomenologischer Sicht" [1972]—[Source given as "Vortragsmanuskript; Erstveröffentlichung"]: pp. 295-308.
"Beispiele für den Einfluß einer Psychotherapie auf die religiöse Einstellung von Analysanden: [1966]": pp. 309-325.
"Modell und Antimodell in der psychosomatischen Medizin" [1967]: pp. 327-346.
"Schizophrenes Kranksein im Lichte einer daseinsanalytischen Phänomenologie" [1975]: pp. 347-372.
"Sexualität und Psychotherapie" [1978]—[Source given as "Vortragsmanuskript; Erstveröffentlichung": pp. 373-386.
"Sigmund Freud und die naturwissenschaftliche Denkmethode" [1973]: pp. 387-404.
"Die psycho-somatische Medizin und das Kausalitätsprinzip" [1974]: pp. 405-422
"Psychotherapie und Wissenschaft" [1974]—[Source given as "Vortragsmanuskript; Erstveröffentlichung"]: pp. 423-442.
"Das Träumen und das Geträumte in daseinsanalytischer Sicht" [excerpts from *Es träumte mir vergangene Nacht...* (Bern: Huber, 1975; 2nd ed. 1991)] [1975]: pp. 443-468.
"Der psychotherapeutische Prozeß" [1977]—[Source given as "Vortragsmanuskript; Erstveröffentlichung"; but see "Der psychotherapeutische Prozeß," in M. Boss, G. Condrau, and A. Hicklin

(eds.), *Leiben und Leben. Beiträge zur Psychosomatik und Psychotherapie* (Bern: Benteli, 1977, pp. 233-346)]: pp. 469-476.
"Die Ontogenese des Menschen—aus der Sicht des Daseinsanalytikers" [1977]: pp. 477-482.

13. *Von der Spannweite der Seele. Ausgewählte Vorträge und Aufsätze aus den Anwendungsbereichen des daseinsanalytischen Menschenverständnisses* (Bern: Benteli, 1982).
[*On the wingspan of the soul. Selected lectures and essays from areas of application of the existential- analytical understanding of man*]

Contents:
"Ist die Psychotherapie rational oder rationell?" ["Das Irrationale in der psychotherapeutischen Behandlung"] [1977]: pp. 9-27.
"Der korrespondierende Wandel von Gesellschaftsqualität und Nuerosenformer im XX.Jahrhundert" [1974]: pp. 28-45.
"Angst und christliches Vertrauen" ["Angst und Gelassenheit im daseinsanalytischer Sicht"] [1981]: pp. 46-60.
"Sprache und Angst im technifizierten Zeitalter" [1981]: pp. 61-68.
"Begegnung mit sich selbst in der Schuld und im Gewissen" [1981]: pp. 69-97.
"Gewähren und Versagen in der Psychotherapie" [1978]: pp. 98-110.
"Das Konzept des Widerstandes in der Daseinsanalyse (in Zusammenarbeit mit Alice Holzhey-Kunz" [1981]: pp. 111-131.
"Das Unbewußte—was ist es?" [1981]: pp. 132-150.
"Triebwelt und Personalisation" [1981]: pp. 151-172.
"Der Einstieg der 'Daseinsanalytik' in das Denken der Ärtze" [1981]: pp. 173-181. [Original version of a text published with Gion Condrau as "Die Weiterentwicklung der Daseinsanalyse nach Ludwig Binswanger."]
"Abriss der Psychotherapie-Entwicklung im 20.Jahrhundert" ["Die Entwicklung der Psychotherapie im 20. Jahrhundert"] [1980]: pp. 182-198.
"Die Bedeutung Martin Heideggers für die Arbeit mit leidenden Menschen und für das Selbstverständnis der Psychotherapie" [1981]: pp. 199-210.
"Dank an Martin Heidegger—Ein Hinweis auf seine Zollikoner Seminare" [1977]: pp. 211-225.

II. EDITED BOOK

14. Martin Heidegger, *Zollikoner Seminare, Protokolle–Gespräche– Briefe* (Frankfurt: Klostermann, 1987; 2nd ed., 1994; 3rd ed., 2006).
  [*Zollikon seminars: protocols, conversations, letters*]

   [Italian translation: *Seminari di Zollikon* (Naples: Guida, 1987)]
   [Japanese translation: *Tsuorikōn zemināru* (Tokyo: Misuzu Shobo, 1991, 1997)]
   [English translation: *Zollikon Seminars: Protocols– Conversations–Letters* (Evanston: Northwestern University Press, 2001)] See (Franz Mayr and Richard Askay)
   [Portuguese translation: *Seminários de Zollikon* (Sao Paulo: Editora Vozes, 2001; 3rd rev. ed., 2017)]
   [Spanish translation: *Seminarios de Zollikon protocolos, diálogos, cartas* (Michoacán: Red Utopia, 2007)]
   [French translation: *Séminaires de Zürich* (Paris: Presses Universitaires, 2010)].
   [Korean translation: 졸리콘 세미나 (2016)]

   [Russian translation: Tsollikonovskie seminary: komentarii i interpretatsii : sbornik nauchnykh rabot
   (Minsk : Logvinaŭ, 2017)].

   [Note: The Heidegger *Gesamtausgabe* (Frankfurt: Klosterman, 2018) edition (volume 89, edited by Peter Trawny) contains reprints of the seminar protocols included in Boss (1989) and Heidegger's notes for the seminars.]

III. CO-EDITED BOOKS

15. *Third International Congress of Psychotherapy* [Zürich 1954] (M. Boss, H. Fierz and B. Stokvis, eds.) (New York: Karger, 1955).

16. *Leiben und Leben* (M. Boss, G. Condrau and A. Hicklin, eds.) (Bern: Berteli, 1977).
   [*Being alive and living life*]

Contents:
"Die psychosomatische Medizin in Nöten" [1955]: pp. 11-18.
"Die notwendige Revolution im ärtzlichen Denken" [1970]: pp. 19-36.
"Das Verhältnis von Leib und Seele im Lichte der Daseinsanalytik" [1977]. Reprinted in *Von Psychoanalyse zur Daseinsanalyse* (Vienna: Europaverlag, 1979, pp. 199-210): pp. 37-70.
[G. Condrau: "Philosophisch-wissenschaftliches Menschenverständnis und ärtzliches Handeln in daseinsanalytischer Sicht"] [1977]: pp. 71-78.
[G. Condrau: "Psychosomatik und Psychotherapie"—I. "Die Grundlagen einer psychosomatischen Medizin" (pp. 81-131); II. Möglichkeiten und Grenzen der Psychotherapie psychosomatischer Krankheiten" (pp. 131-210)] [1977]: pp. 79-210.
[G. Condrau: "Psychotherapie und Krankenlassen"] [1977]: pp. 211-226.
"Die daseinsgemäße Betrachtungsweise und die psychotherapeutische Beeinflußbarkeit menschlicher Körperleiden" [1977]: pp. 227-232.
"Der psychotherapeutische Prozeß: [1977]. Reprinted in *Von Psychoanalyse zur Daseinsanalyse* (Vienna: Europaverlag, 1979), pp. 199-210: pp. 233-246.
[A. Hicklin: "Die gesellschaftspolitische Bedeutung der psychosomatischen Medizin"] [1977]: pp. 246-26
[A. Hicklin: "Die Therapie einer jungen Frau mit schweren neurotischen und psychosomatischen Störungen"] [1977]: pp. 261-338.

IV. CHAPTERS IN BOOKS

17. "Indications et effets de la cure de sommeil," in *Comptes rendus. Congrès des médecins alienistes et neurologistes de pays de la langue française* (Paris: Masson, 1936), pp. 1-4.
    [Indications and effects of the sleep cure]

18. "Psychotherapeutischer Beitrag zur Schizophrenielehre," in *Second International Congress of Psychiatry* (Basel: Karger, 1957), Volume 3, pp. 254-259.
    [A psychotherapeutic contribution to the theory of schizophrenia]

[English translation: "The Role of Psychotherapy in Schizophrenia," in *Indian Journal of Psychiatry* 1(1), 1958, pp. 1-9.] (B)

19. "Warum verhält sich der Mensch überhaupt sozial?," in *Proceedings of the Third World Congress of Psychiatry* [Montreal, June 9, 1961] (Montreal: McGill University Press, 1961), Volume 1, pp. 228-233.
[Why does man behave socially at all?]

[English translation: "What Makes Us Behave at All Socially?," in *Review of Existential Psychology and Psychiatry* 4(1), 1964, pp. 53-68]. [Lecture given in English at Harvard University, July 23, 1963.] (B)

20. "Psychosomatics and Existentialism," in *Proceedings of the Third World Congress of Psychiatry* [Montreal, June 4-10, 1961] (Montreal: McGill University Press, 1961), Volume 3, pp. 277-280. (B)
[Psychosomatics and existentialism]

21. "Vorwort" to Carlos Seguín, *Der Artz und sein Patient* (Bern: Huber, 1965), pp. 7-18. See 1965d.
[Preface to Carlos Seguin, *The doctor and his patient*]

[English translation: "Introduction" to Carlos Alberto Seguín, *Love and Psychotherapy. The Psychotherapeutic Eros* (New York: Libra, 1965), pp. v-xiv.] (B)

22. "Martin Heidegger und die Ärzte," in G. Neske (ed.), *Martin Heidegger zum 70. Geburtstag* (Neske: Pfullingen, 1959), pp. 276-290. Adapted version printed in *Von der Psychoanalyse zur Daseinsanalyse* (Vienna: Europaverlag, 1979, pp. 203-244.
[Martin Heidegger and the doctors]

23. "Foreword" [1970] to Govind Kaul, *Govind Amrit* (Bombay: Prithwinath Niranjannath Pandit, 1975), pp. 1-2.
[Foreword to *Govind Amrit*]

24. "Entmythologisierung der psychosomatischen Medizin," in J. Lassner (ed.), *Hypnosis and Psychosomatic Medicine* (New York: Springer, 1967), pp. 35-53. Reprinted in *Zeitschrift für klinische Psychologie und Psychotherapie* 25(2), 1977, pp. 136-151.
[Demythologization of psychosomatic medicine]

25. "Medard Boss," in L. Pongratz (ed.), *Psychotherapie in Selbstdarstellungen* (Bern: Huber, 1973), pp. 71-106.
[Medard Boss]

[English translation: "Medard Boss," *Existential Analysis* 30(1), pp. 169-198. (Miles Groth)

26. "Der korrespondierende Wandel von Gesellschaftsqualität und Neurosenformen im 20.Jahrhundert," in G. Condrau and A. Hicklin (eds.), *Individuum, Familie, Gesellschaft im Spannungsfeld zwischen Zwang und Freiheit* [*Weiterentwicklung der Psychoanalyse und ihrer Anwendungen* 6] (Zürich: Vandenhoeck and Ruprecht, 1974), pp. 153-167. Reprinted in *Von der Spannweite der Seele. Ausgewählte Vorträge und Aufsätze aus den Anwendungsbereichen des daseinsanalytischen Menschenverständnisses* (Bern: Benteli, 1982), pp. 28-45.
[Corresponding changes in the quality of social life and the forms of neurosis in the 20th century]

27. "Solitude et communauté," in G. Balandier *et al.* (ed.), *Solitude et Communication. Rencontres Internationales de Genève* (Neuchatel: Edition de la Baconnière, 1975), pp. 47-68.
[Solitude and community]
[Portuguese translation: "Solidao e comunidade," in *Daseinsanalyse* (Sao Paulo) **2**, 1976, pp. 25-45].
[German translation: "Einsamkeit und Gemeinschaft," in *Daseinsanalyse* **1**(1) (Zürich), 1984, pp. 6-22.

28. "Das Träumen und das Geträumte in daseinsanalytischer Sicht," in R. Battegay and A.Trenkel (eds.), *Der Traum* (Bern: Huber, 1976), pp. 71-93. Reprinted in *Von der Psychoanalyse zur Daseinsanalyse* (Vienna: Europaverlag, 1979), pp. 443-468. Includes excerpts from *Es träumte mir vergangene Nacht...* (Bern: Huber, 1975; 2nd ed. 1991).
[Dreams and the dreamed from the existential-analytical perspective]

[English translation: "Dreaming and the Dreamed in the Daseinsanalytic Way of Seeing," in *Soundings* 60(3), 1977, pp. 235-263.] (Tom Cook)

29. **"Flight from Death—Mere Survival; and Flight into Death—Suicide,"** in B. Wolman (ed.), *Between Survival and Suicide* (New York: Gardner Press, 1976), pp. 1-24. (B)
[Flight from death—mere survival and flight into death—suicide]

30. "Die Ontogenese des Menschen—aus der Sicht des Daseinsanalytikers," in G. Condrau and A. Hicklin (eds.), *Das Werden des Menschen* (Bern: Benteli, 1977), pp. 105-119. Reprinted in *Von der Psychoanalyse zur Daseinsanalyse* (Vienna: Europaverlag, 1979), pp. 483-490.
[The ontogenesis of man ... from the perspective of the existential analyst]

31. "Die daseinsgemäße Betrachtungsweise und die psychotherapeutische Beeinflußbarkeit menschlicher Körperleiden," in M. Boss, G. Condrau, and A. Hicklin (eds.), *Leiben und Leben. Beiträge zur Psychosomatik und Psychotherapie* (Bern: Berteli, 1977), pp. 227-232.
[The existentially informed approach and psychotherapeutic suggestibility in human physical ailments]

32. "Der psychotherapeutische Prozeß," in M. Boss, G. Condrau, and A. Hicklin (eds.), *Leiben und Leben. Beiträge zur Psychosomatik und Psychotherapie* (Bern: Berteli, 1977), pp. 233-346, and in *Von der Psychoanalyse zur Daseinsanalyse. Wege zu einem neuen Selbstverständnis* (Vienna: Europaverlag, 1979), pp. 469-476.
[The psychotherapeutic process]

33. "Schlußwort" in F. Töpfer (ed.), *Verstümmung oder Selbstverwirklichung? Die Boss-Mitscherlich-Kontroverse* (Olton: Walter Verlag, 1981; Stuttgart: Bad Cannstatt, 2012), pp. 95-104.
[Closing remarks (Conference on the Boss-Mitscherlich controversy)]

34. "Dank an Martin Heidegger–Ein Hinweis auf seine Zollikoner Seminare," in G. Neske (ed.), *Erinnerung an Martin Heidegger* (Pfullingen: Neske, 1977), pp. 31-45. Reprinted in *Von der Spannweite der Seele. Ausgewählte Vorträge und Aufsätze aus den Anwendungsbereichen des daseinsanalytischen Menschenverständnisses* (Bern: Benteli, 1982), pp. 211-225.
[Thanks to Martin Heidegger. A note on his Zollikon seminars]

[English translation: "Martin Heidegger's Zollikon Seminars," in *Review of Existential Psychology and Psychiatry* 16(1-3), 1978-79, pp. 7-20.] (Brian Kenny)

35. "Existential Analysis," in B. Wolman (ed.), *International Encyclopedia of Psychiatry, Psychology, Psychoanalysis and Neurology* (New York: Aesculapius, 1977), pp. 395-400. (B)
[Existential analysis]

36. "Widersprochener Widerspruch," in G. Condrau and A. Hicklin (eds.), *Der Mensch: Gegenstand der Naturwissenschaft?* (Bern: Benteli, 1978), pp. 41-50.
[Contradiction contradicted]

37. "Das Sein zum Tode in tiefenpsychologischer Sicht," in G. Condrau (ed.), *Transzendenz, Imagination und Kreativität. Die Psychologie des 20.Jahrhunderts* [Volume 15] (Zürich: Kindler, 1979), pp. 454-463.
[Being-towards-death from the perspective of depth psychology]

38. "Das Irrationale in der psychotherapeutischen Behandlung," in G. Condrau (ed.), *Transzendenz, Imagination und Kreativität* (Zürich: Kindler, 1979), pp. 687-696. Reprinted as "Ist die Psychotherpie rational oder rationell?," in *Von der Spannweite der Seele. Ausgewählte Vorträge und Aufsätze aus den Anwendungsbereichen des daseinsanalytischen Menschenverständnisses* (Bern: Benteli, 1982), pp, pp. 9-27.
[The irrational in psychotherapeutic practice]

[English translation: "Is Psychotherapy Rational or Rationalistic?," in *Review of Existential Psychology and Psychiatry* 19(2-3), 1984-85, pp. 115-127.] (E.S. Goodstein)

39. "Martin Heidegger und seine Bedeutung für die gesellschaftliche Evolution," in A. Hicklin (ed.), *Wandel und Tradition* (Bern: Benteli, 1980), pp. 111-129. Adapted version reprinted in *Von Psychoanalyse zur Daseinsanalyse* (Vienna: Europaverlag, 1979), pp. 199-210.
[Martin Heidegger and his significance for the evolution of society]

40. "Begegnung und Auseinandersetzung mit sich selbst in der Schuld und im Gewissen," in R. Battegay (ed.), *Herausforderung und*

Begegnung in der Psychiatrie [Festschrift zum 60.Geburtstag von G. Benedetti] (Bern: Hans Huber, 1981), pp. 54-60. Reprinted in *Von der Spannweite der Seele. Ausgewählte Vorträge und Aufsätze aus den Anwendungsbereichen des daseinsanalytischen Menschenverständnisses* (Bern: Benteli, 1982), pp. 69-97.
[Encounter and self-confrontation in guilt and in conscience]

41. "Triebwelt und Personalisation," in H. Böckle, F.K. Kaufmann, K. Rahner, and B. Welte (eds.), *Christlicher Glaube in moderner Welt* (Freiburg: Herder, 1981), Volume 6, pp. 8-27. Reprinted in *Von der Spannweite der Seele. Ausgewählte Vorträge und Aufsätze aus den Anwendungsbereichen des daseinsanalytischen Menschenverständnisses* (Bern: Benteli, 1982), pp. 151-172.
[The world of drives and personalization]

[Spanish translation: "Mundo pulsional y personalizacíon," in H.Döring (ed.), *Experiencia de la contingencia y pregunta por el sentido* (Madrid, SM, 1985)]

42. "Angst und Gelassenheit im daseinsanalytischer Sicht," in H. Böckle, F.K. Kaufmann, K. Rahner, and B. Welte (eds.), *Christlicher Glaube in moderner Welt* (Freiburg: Herder, 1981), Volume 9, pp. 69-85. Reprinted as "Angst und christliche Vertrauen," in *Von der Spannweite der Seele. Ausgewählte Vorträge und Aufsätze aus den Anwendungsbereichen des daseinsanalytischen Menschenverständnisses* (Bern: Benteli, 1982), pp. 46-60.
[Anxiety and composure from the existential-analytical perspective]

43. "Wirklichkeit als das Sich-Entbergen von Seiendem," in E. Grassi and H. Schmale (eds.), *Das Gespräch als Ereignis* (Munich: Fink, 1982), pp. 99-108.
[Actuality as the self-revelation of what is there]

44. **"A Phenomenological Approach to Sexual Perversions," in A. de Koning and F. Jenner (eds.), Phenomenology and Psychiatry (New York: Academic Press, 1982), pp. 85-95. (B)**
[A phenomenological approach to sexual perversions]

45. "Interpretaçao daseinsanalítica dos sonhos," in G. Lopes (ed.), *Progressos en terapeutica psiquiátrica* (Porto: Biblioteca do Hospital do Conde de Ferreira, 1982), pp. 335-346.
[The existential-analytical interpretation of dreams]

46. "Anstöße Martin Heideggers für eine andere Psychiatrie," in H.-H. Gander (ed.), *Von Heidegger her. Meßkirchner Vorträge* (Frankfurt: Klostermann, 1991), pp. 125-140.
[Martin Heidegger's initiatives for a different kind of psychiatry]

47. **"Preface to the American Translation of Martin Heidegger's *Zollikon Seminars*," in Martin Heidegger, *Zollikon Seminars. Protocols—Conversations—Letters*** (Evanston: Northwestern University Press, 2001), pp. ix-xii. (B).
[Preface to Martin Heidegger, *Zollikon Seminars. Protocols—Conversations—Letters*]

[Note: The text is dated Spring 1989. Boss died on December 21, 1990 before completing the preface. His widow, Marianne Boss-Linsmayer, completed it. According to the translators, it contains a few sentences from her preface to the second German edition (1994) and some concluding words that pertain to the English translation (pp. xi-xii).]

V. JOURNAL ARTICLES

48. "Zur Frage der erbbiologischen Bedeutung des Alkohols," in *Monatschrift* für Psychiatrie und Neurologie **72**, 1929, pp. 264-292. This was Boss's dissertation, supervised by Hans W. Meier, that gained him the title "Dr. med." following his completion of the MD degree.
[On the question of the evolutionary biological significance of alcohol]

49. "Psychologisch-charakterologische Untersuchungen bei antisozialen Psychopathen mit Hilfe des Rorschach'schen Formdeutversuches," in *Zeitschrfit für gesamte Neurologie und Psychiatrie* **133**, 1931, pp. 544- 575.
[Psychological and characterological investigations of antisocial psychopaths using the Rorschach Inkblot Test]

50. "Halluzinationen *in statu nascendi*," in *Schweizer Archive für Neurologie und Psychiatrie* **32**(2), 1933, pp. 1- 4.
[Hallucinations in process of formation]

51. "Die psychischen Energieverschiebungen im Verlaufe eines schizophrenen Schubes," in *Schweizer Archive für Neurologie und Psychiatrie* **36**(1), 1935, pp. 58-62.
[Psychic energy displacements in the course of a schizophrenic episode]

52. "Die psychische Dynamik der Schlafkur bei Schizophrenien," in *Schweizer Archive für Neurologie und Psychiatrie* **36**(2), 1935, pp. 209-220.
[The psychodynamics of the sleep cure in schizophrenics]

53. "Die Grundprinzipien der Schizophrenietherapie im historischen Rückblick," in *Zeitschrfit für gesamte Neurologie und Psychiatrie* **157**(3), 1937, pp. 358-392. Reprinted in *Von der Psychoanalyse zur Daseinsanalyse* (Vienna: Europaverlag, 1979), pp.11-53.
[Historical review of the fundamental principles of the therapy of schizophrenia]

54. "Individuelle Vorbehandlung zur kollektiven Arbeitstherapie bei schweren, chronischen Schizophrenen," in *Schweizer Archive für Neurologie und Psychiatrie* **62**(1), 1938, pp. 15-26. Reprinted in *Von der Psychoanalyse zur Daseinsanalyse* (Vienna: Europaverlag, 1979), pp. 55-70.
[Preparation of individuals with severe chronic schizophrenia for group occupational therapy]

55. "Psychopathologie des Traumes bei schizophrenen und organischen Psychosen," in *Zeitschrfit für gesamte Neurologie und Psychiatrie* **162**(3), 1938, pp. 459-494.
[The psychopathology of dreams in schizophrenic and organic psychoses]

56. "Über drei Kategorien vermeidbarer Mißerfolge in der ärztlichen Allgemeinpraxis," in *Schweizerische medizinische Wochenschrift* **69**(26), 1939, pp. 602-607. Reprinted in *Von der Psychoanalyse zur Daseinsanalyse* (Vienna: Europaverlag, 1979), pp. 71-93.
[On three categories of avoidable failures in general medical practice]

57. "Kleine und große Psychotherapie," in *Schweizerische medizinische Wochenschrift* **70**(6), 1940, pp. 113-126.
    [Brief and intensive psychotherapy]

58. "Über die geheimen Mühsale seelischen Gesundseins und ihre Linderung," in *Gesundheit und Wohlfahrt* **9/10**, 1940, pp. 581-587.
    [On the hidden challenges to psychological well-being and their mitigation]

59. "Die funktionellen Schlafstörungen in der Schizophrenie," in *Schweizerische medizinische Wochenschrift* **71**(12), 1941, pp. 390- 391.
    [Functional disturbances of sleep in schizophrenia]

60. "Nahrungsmittelrationierung und Volkspsychologie," in *Gesundheit und Wohlfahrt* **11**, 1941, pp. 1-8.
    [Food rationing and popular psychology]

61. "Psychohygiene in vorderer Linie (Militärpsychiatrie)," in *Schweizerische medizinische Wochenschrift* **71**(23), 1941, pp. 707-711.
    [Psychological health on the front lines (military psychiatry)]

62. "Alte und neue Schocktherapien und Schocktherapeuten," in *Zeitschrfit für gesamte Neurologie und Psychiatrie* **173**, 1941, pp. 776-782. Reprinted in *Von der Psychoanalyse zur Daseinsanalyse* (Vienna: Europaverlag, 1979), pp. 95-103.
    [Early and recent electroshock therapies and electroshock therapists]

63. "Die Funktion der psychiatrischen Beratungsstelle in den selbständigen Heereseinheiten," in *Vierteljahresschrift für Schweizerische Sanitätsoffiziere* **21**(2), 1944, pp. 85-90.
    [The function of the psychiatric counseling center in independent army units]

64. "*Enuresis nocturna*," in *Schweizerische medizinische Wochenschrift* **75**(14), 1945, pp. 293-305.
    [Bed-wetting]

65. "Vom Weg und Ziel der tiefenpsychologischen Therapie," in *Psyche* **1**(3), 1948, pp. 321-339. Reprinted in *Von der Psychoanalyse zur Daseinsanalyse* (Vienna: Europaverlag, 1979), pp. 123-144.
    [The method and goal of depth-psychological therapy]

66. "Die Möglichkeiten und Grenzen der Psychotherapie," in *Schweizerische Zeitschrift für Psychologie und ihre Anwendungen* **7**(4), 1948, pp. 252-268. Reprinted in *Von der Psychoanalyse zur Daseinsanalyse* (Vienna: Europaverlag, 1979), pp. 105-121.
    [The possibilities and limits of psychotherapy]

67. "Die Blutdruckkrankheiten als menschliches Problem," in *Psyche* **2**(4), 1949, pp. 499-517.
    [Blood pressure ailments as a human problem]

68. "Die Grundlagen einer psychosomatischen Medizin," in *Schweizerische medizinische Wochenschrift* **79**(50), 1950, pp. 1203-1208.
    [Fundamentals of psychosomatic medicine]

69. "Erwiderung. Zum Bericht über mein Referat auf der 66. Wanderversammlung der südwestdeutschen Psychiater und Neurologen in Badenweiler," in *Psyche* **4**(7), 1950, pp. 394-400. Reprinted as "Erwiderung. Zum Bericht über mein Referat auf der 66. Wanderversammlung der südwestdeutschen Psychiater und Neurologen in Badenweiler," in F. Töpfer (ed.), *Verstümmung oder Selbstverwirklichung? Die Boss-Mitscherlich-Kontroverse* (Olton: Walter Verlag, 1981; Stuttgart: Bad Cannstatt, 2012), pp. 19-28. Participants in the discussion included Carl Gustav Jung, Manfred Bleuler, Ludwig Binswanger, Viktor von Weizäcker.
    [Reply to the report on my presentation at the 66th gathering of Southwest German psychiatrists and neurologists held in Badenweiler (Conference on the Boss-Mitscherlich controversy)]

70. "Die neuesten Fortschritte auf dem Gebiete der Psychoanalyse," in *Studium Generale* **3**(6), 1950, pp. 303-308.
    [Latest advances in the field of psychoanalysis]

71. "Beitrag zur daseinsanalytischen Fundierung des psychiatrischen Denkens," in *Schweizer Archive für Neurologie und Psychiatrie* **67**(1), 1951, pp. 15-19. Reprinted in *Von der Psychoanalyse zur Daseinsanalyse* (Vienna: Europaverlag, 1979), pp. 145-150.
    [Contribution to the existential-analytical foundation of psychiatric thinking]

72. "Erfahrungen mit dem neuen Schlafmittel 'Plexonal' (Sandoz)," in *Praxis* **40**(33), 1951, pp. 679-683.
[Experiences with the hypnotic Plexonal [Scopolamine] (Sandoz)]

73. "Mensch und Technik in der heutigen Medizin," in *Schweizerische medizinische Wochenschrift* **82**(25), 1952, pp. 653-657.
[Man and technology in today's medicine]

    [English translation: "Mechanistic and Holistic Thinking in Modern Medicine," in *American Journal of Psychoanalysis* 14(1), 1954, pp. 48-54.] (B)

74. "Die Bedeutung der Daseinsanalyse für die Psychologie und die Psychiatrie," in *Psyche* **6**(3), 1952, pp. 178-186. Reprinted in *Von der Psychoanalyse zur Daseinsanalyse* (Vienna: Europaverlag, 1979), pp. 151-160.
[The significance of existential analysis for psychology and psychiatry]

75. "Über Herkunft und Wesen der tiefenpsychologischen Archetypus-Begriffes," in *Psyche* **6**(10), 1953, pp. 584-597.
[On the origin and essence of the depth-psychological concept of the archetype]

76. "Wie soll eine Frigidität in der Praxis beurteilt und behandelt werden?," in *Deutsche medizinische Wochenschrift* **78**(45), 1953, pp. 1573-1576.
[How should frigidity be evaluated and treated in practice?]

    [Italian translation: "Come considerare e trattare la frigidità?," in *Medicina Psicosomatica* **1**, 1956, pp. 9-12].

77. "Reglementierung der Tätigkeit nicht-ärztlicher Psychologen," in *Schweizerische Ärzte-Zeitung* **34**, 1953, pp. 272-275.
[Regulation of the activity of non-medical psychologists]

78. "Grundsätzliches zur Wissenschaftlichkeit der Traumbedeutung," in *Schweizerische Zeitschrift für Psychologie und ihre Anwendungen* **13**(2), 1954, pp. 128-135.
[Basics of the scientific nature of dream interpretation]

79. "Die psychosomatische Medizin in Nöten," in *Medizin Heute* **4**(4), 1955, pp. 185-187. Reprinted in M. Boss, G. Condrau and A. Hicklin (eds.), *Leiben und Leben. Beiträge zur Psychosomatik und Psychotherapie* (Bern: Benteli, 1977), pp. 11-18.
[Psychosomatic medicine in distress]

80. **"Moreno's 'Existentialism, Daseinanalyse and Psychodrama': A Discussion," *International Journal of Sociometry and Sociatry* 1, 1956, pp. 111-113. (B)**
[Moreno's "Existentialism, Daseinanalyse and psychodrama": A discussion]

81. "Daseinsanalytik und Psychotherapie. Über die Grenzen der Psychoanalyse," in *Deutsche Universitätszeitung* **11**(23-24), 1956, pp. 17-19.
[Analytics of existence and psychotherapy. On the limits of psychoanalysis]

[English translation: "'Daseinsanalysis' and Psychotherapy," in J. Masserman and J.L. Moreno (eds.), *Progress in Psychotherapy. Volume II. Anxiety and Therapy* (New York: Grune and Stratton, 1957), pp. 156-161. Reprinted in H. Ruitenbeek (ed.) *Psychoanalysis and Existential Philosophy* (New York: Dutton, 1962), pp. 81-89.] (B)

82. "Wirkungsweise und Indikation der Psychotherapie," in *Schweizerische medizinische Wochenschrift* **87**(6), 1957, pp. 128-133.
[The mechanism of action and indications for psychotherapy]

[Italian translation: "Modo d'agire e indicazioni della psicoterapia," in *Medicina Psicosomatica* **3**(1), 1958, pp. 3-17].

83. "Zusammenfassung und Schlußwort zum internationalen Symposium über die Psychotherapie der Schizophrenie," in *Acta psychotherapeutica et Psychosomatica et Orthopaedagogica* **5**(2-4), 1957, pp. 352-359.
[Summary and closing remarks at the international symposium on the psychotherapy of schizophrenia (Lausanne 1957)]

84. "Die Psychotherapie des praktischen Arztes," in *Schweizerische medizinische Wochenschrift* **89**(51), 1959, pp. 1336-1341. Reprinted

in *Von der Psychoanalyse zur Daseinsanalyse* (Vienna: Europaverlag, 1979), pp. 187-202.
[Psychotherapy for the practicing physician]

85. "Kleine und große Psychotherapie der essentiellen Hypertoniker," in *Acta Psychosomatica* **3**, 1959, pp. 9-40.
[Brief and intensive psychotherapy for essential hypertension]

[French translation: 'Petite' Psychothérapie et 'Grande' Psychothérapie des Hypertendus Essentiels (Basel: Geigy, 1959].

86. "Psicoanálisis y análisis del 'dasein,'" in *Revista de Psiquiatría y Psicología médica de Europa y América Latina* **4**(1), 1959, pp. 20-26.
[Psychoanalysis and the analytics of 'existence']

[French translation: "Psychanalyse et analyse du 'dasein,'" in *Acta Psychotherapeutica et Psychosomatica* **8**(3), 1960, pp. 161-171].

87. "Große Psychotherapie der psychosomatischen Krankheiten," in *Schweizerische medizinische Wochenschrift* **90**(8), 1960, pp. 173-177.
[The intensive psychotherapy of psychosomatic diseases]

88. "Das Ich? Die Motivation?" in *Schweizerische Zeitschrift für Psychologie und ihre Anwendungen* **19**(4), 1960, pp. 299-306.
[Paper read at the 11th International Congress of Psychology, Bonn, August 2, 1960.]
[The I? Motivation?]

[French translation: "Le problème du moi dans la motivation," in *L'évolution Psychiatrique* **25**(4), 1960, pp. 481-489.
[English translation: "Ego? Motivation?" in *Journal of Existentialism* 1, 1960, pp. 275-283. Reprinted as "The Ego? Human Motivation?" in *Acta Psychologica* 19, 1961, pp. 217-222.] (B)

89. **"Letter to Heidegger of [January 12, 1960]"** (1960), in *Review of Existential Psychology and Psychiatry* 27(1-3), 2002-2003, pp. 37-39. Reprinted as a monograph by Keith Hoeller (ed.), *The Heidegger-Boss Relationship* (Seattle: Review of Existential Psychology and Psychiatry, 2008), pp. 37-39. (Eva Mader)
[Letter to Heidegger, January 12, 1960]

90. "Daseinsanalytische Bemerkungen zu Freuds Vorstellung des 'Unbewußten,'" in *Zeitschrift für psychosomatische Medizin* **7**, 1960-61, pp. 130-141. Reprinted in *Von der Psychoanalyse zur Daseinsanalyse* (Vienna: Europaverlag, 1979), pp. 245-266.
[Existential-analytical remarks on Freud's concept of the 'unconscious']

91. "Die Bedeutung der Daseinsanalyse für die psychoanalytische Praxis," in *Zeitschrift für psychosomatische Medizin* **7**, 1960-61, pp. 162-171. Reprinted in *Von der Psychoanalyse zur Daseinsanalyse* (Vienna: Europaverlag, 1979), pp. 267-285.
[The significance of existential analysis for psychoanalytic practice]

92. **"Outline of the Analysis of Dasein," in *Philosophical Bulletin. Visva Tattvajnana Mandira Quarterly* 1(1), 1962, pp. 49-64. (B)**
[Outline of the analysis of *Dasein*]

93. **"The Conception of Man in Natural Science and Daseinsanalysis," in *Comprehensive Psychiatry* 3(4), August 1962, pp. 193-214.** (H.A. Frey)
[The conception of man in natural science and daseinsanalysis]

94. "Gedanken über eine schizophrene Halluzination," in *Schweizer Archive für Neurologie und Psychiatrie* **91**(1), 1963, pp. 87-95.
[Thoughts on a schizophrenic hallucination]

95. **"Presidential Address at the Opening Session [of the VIth International Congress of Psychotherapy, August 24-29, 1964]," in *Psychotherapy and Psychosomatics* 13(1-3), 1965, pp. xii-xii. (B)**
[President's opening address, August 24, 1964. VIth International congress of psychotherapy]

96. **"Presidential Address at the Closing Session [of the VIth International Congress of Psychotherapy, August 24-29, 1964]," in *Psychotherapy and Psychosomatics* 13(1-3), 1965, pp. 246-248. (B)**
[President's closing address, August 29, 1964. VIth International congress of psychotherapy]

97. **"Discussion of [the] Paper by J. Ruesch [August 24-29, 1964, London]"**, in *Psychotherapy and Psychosomatics* 13(1-3), 1965, pp. 82-86. (B)
    [Discussion of Ruesch, August 1964]

    [Note: The Sixth International Congress of Psychotherapy, London 1964, featured papers given by, among others, Michael Fordham, Anna Freud, and R.D. Laing. Boss's opening and closing remarks are included.]

98. "Begegnung in der Psychotherapie," in *Psychotherapy and Psychosomatics* 13(5), 1965, pp. 332-341. Reprinted in *Von der Psychoanalyse zur Daseinsanalyse* (Vienna: Europaverlag, 1979), pp. 287-294. [Source given as "Vortragsmanuskript [lecture manuscript]"]. Presented on May 1, 1964, in Milan, at a roundtable on therapeutic encounter for the Milan Group for the Advancement of Psychotherapy. An Italian transcript of Boss's comments and his replies to comments by the other panelists, Gaetano Benedetti and Eugène Minkowski, was published in *Psicoterapia e Scienze Umane* (Milan) 51(2), 2017, pp. 267-284. Sections of the lecture were printed in Boss's "Introduction" to Carlos Alberto Seguín's *Love and Psychotherapy. The Therapeutic Eros* and the German version of the book. See 1965e.
    [Encounter in psychotherapy]

99. "Cinco lecciones de introduccion a la analitica del dasein," in *Cuadernos de Psiquiatría* 3(4), 1966, pp. 17-38.
    [Five introductory lectures on the analytics of existence]

100. "Beispiele für den Einfluß einer Psychotherapie auf die religiöse Einstellung von Analysanden," in *Theologia practica. Zeitschrift für Praktische Theologue und Religionspädagogik* 1(3), 1966, pp. 222-234. Reprinted in *Von der Psychoanalyse zur Daseinsanalyse* (Vienna: Europaverlag, 1979), pp. 309-325, and as "Der Einfluß der Daseinsanalyse auf die Religiosität der Analysand," in G. Condrau (ed.), *Transzendenz, Imagination und Kreativität* (Zürich: Kindler, 1979), pp. 321-329.
    [Evidence for the influence of psychotherapy on the religious attitude of the analysand]

101. "Modell und Antimodell in der psychosomatischen Medizin," in *Therapeutische Umschau* **24**, 1967, pp. 536-545. Reprinted in *Von der Psychoanalyse zur Daseinsanalyse* (Vienna: Europaverlag, 1979) [1937-1978], pp. 327-346. Reply to a presentation by F. Meerwein, "Psychosomatsche Modellvorstellung" (May 27, 1967, Zürich University Psychiatric Clinic), in *Therapeutische Umschau* **24**, 1967, pp. 343-351.
    [Paradigm and counterparadigm in psychosomatic medicine]

102. **"Conversation with Mary Harrington Hall," in *Psychology Today* 2(7), December 1968, pp. 58-65.**
    [Conversation with Mary Harrington]

103. "Der Mensch—Gegenstand wissenschaftlicher," in *Psychosomatische Medizin* **1**(1-2), 1968-69, pp. 1-4.
    [Man—an object of science]

104. "Die notwendige Revolution im ärztlichen Denken," in *Therapeutische Umschau* **27**(12), 1970, pp. 783-790. Reprinted in M. Boss, G. Condrau and A. Hicklin (eds.), *Leiben und Leben* (Bern: Berteli, 1977), pp. 19-36.
    [A needed revolution in medical thinking]

105. "Die notwendige Revolution der Weltanschauung," in *Journal der Reisehochschule Zürich und des Reisehochschulclubs Zürichs* **10**, 1971, pp. 1-22. Reprinted in A. Gloor (ed.), *Die Zukunft im Angriff. Die Schweiz auf dem Weg ins 21.Jahrhunderts* (Frauenfeld: Huber, 1971), p. 11-47.
    [A needed revolution in worldview]

106. **"The Training of the Future Psychotherapist. Improvement of Psychiatric Services and Teaching Programs," in *Indian Journal of Psychiatry* 15, 1972, pp. 4-14. (B)**
    [The training of the future psychotherapist. Improvement of psychiatric services and teaching programs]

107. "Sturmzeichen in der Psychologie und Psychiatrie. Epilog zu einem revolutionären Internationalen Psychotherapeuten-Kongress," in *Psychotherapy and Psychosomatics* **20**(1-2), 1972, pp. 92-106.
    [Warning signs of a storm in psychology and psychiatry. Epilogue to a revolutionary international congress on psychotherapy]

108. "Arzt und Tod. Ein daseinsanalytischer Versuch" [1971], in *Psychosomatische Medizin* **4**, 1972, pp. 2-12.
[The physician and death. An existential-analytical investigation]

[Portguese translation: "O Médico e a Morte. Um Ensaio Analítico-Existencial," in *Angústia, culpa e libertação: ensaios de psicanálise existancial* (Saõ Paulo : Livraria Duas Cidades, 1975), pp. 67-77. Also contains a translation of "Sturmzeichen in der Psychologie und Psychiatrie. Epilog zu einem revolutionären Internationalen Psychotherapeuten-Kongress," in *Psychotherapy and Psychosomatics* **20**(1-2), 1972, pp. 92-106.]

109. "Die Bedeutung der Daseinsanalyse für die Psychiatrie, dargestellt aufgrund der Behandlung einer schizophrenen Psychose," in *Therapeutische Umschau* **30**(1), 1973, pp. 5-11.
[The significance of existential analysis for psychiatry illustrated by the treatment of a schizophrenic psychosis]

110. "Sigmund Freud und die naturwissenschaftliche Denkmethode," in *Hexagon* **1**(1), 1973, pp. 1-7 and **1**(2), 1973, pp. 1-6. Reprinted in *Von der Psychoanalyse zur Daseinsanalyse* (Vienna: Europaverlag, 1979) [1937-1978], pp. 387-404.
[Sigmund Freud and natural scientific method of thinking]

111. "Die psycho-somatische Medizin und das Kausalitätsprinzip," in *Hexagon* **2**(2), 1974, pp. 8-18. Reprinted in *Von der Psychoanalyse zur Daseinsanalyse* (Vienna: Europaverlag, 1979) [1937-1978], pp. 405-422.
[Psycho-somatic medicine and the principle of causality]

112. "El 'estar enfermo' del esquizofrénico entendido desde el analise existencial," in *Acta Psiquiatrica-Psicologica América Latina* **21**(1), 1975, pp. 6-24.
[The schizophrenic's "being ill" understood in terms of existential analysis]

[German translation: "Schizophrenes Kranksein im Lichte einer daseinsanalytischen Phänomenologie," in *Therapeutische Umschau* **33**(7), 1976, pp. 452-464. Reprinted in *Von der Psychoanalyse zur Daseinsanalyse* (Vienna: Europa, 1979) [1937-1978], pp. 347-372]

[Portuguese translation: "O modo de ser esquizofrenico à luz de uma fenomenología daseinanalítica," in *Revista de Associação Médica Brasileira Daseinsanalyse* **3**, 1977, pp. 5-28].

113. "Cultura e psicoterapia," in *Daseinsanalyse* (Sao Paulo) **2**, 1976, pp. 25-44.
[Culture and psychotherapy]

114. "Das Leib-Seele-Problem im Lichte der Daseinsanalyse," in *Psychosomatische Medizin* **6**(3-4), 1976, pp. 106-128. Reprinted in M. Boss, G. Condrau, G. and A. Hicklin (eds), *Leiben und Leben. Beiträge zur Psychosomatik und Psychotherapie* (Bern: Berteli, 1977), pp. 37-70.
[Japanese translation, in Y. Masatoshi (ed.), *Martin Heidegger-Festschrift* (Tokyo: Risosha) **1**, 1975, pp. 120-143.]
[The mind-body problem in light of existential analysis]

115. **"Medard Boss" [Tribute to Martin Heidegger], in Richard Wisser (ed.), *Martin Heidegger in Conversation*, New Delhi: Arnold-Heinemann, 1977, pp. 9-11. The text is based on *Martin Heidegger im Gespräch*, Freiburg: Alber, 1970.** The translator is given as B. Srinivasa Murthy.
[Medard Boss]

116. "Mit dem Terror leben," in *Rheinische Post* **144**, June 25, 1977, p. 8.
[Living with terror]

117. "Erziehung Ja oder Nein?" in *Neue Zürcher Zeitung* **216**, September 15, 1977, p. 46.
[Education—Yes or no?]

118. "Neid entfacht Terror. Das Phänomen menschlicher Gewalttätigkeit," in *Darmstädter Echo* **180**, August 6, 1977, pp. 37-38.
[Envy triggers terror. The phenomenon of human violence]

119. "Der neue Wandel der Neurosen-Erkenntnisse der Psychotherapie," in *Universitas* **33**(10), 1978, pp. 1023-1030.
[Current changes in the identification of the neuroses in psychotherapy]

120. "Sexualität und Psychotherapie," in *Psychosomatische Medizin* **8**(2), 1978, pp. 118-128. Reprinted in *Von der Psychoanalyse zur Daseinsanalyse* (Vienna: Europaverlag, 1979), pp. 373-386.
[Sexuality and psychotherapy]

121. "Das Träumen. Ein Therapeuticum magnum," in *Hexagon* **8**(1), 1980, pp. 15-24.
[Dreaming. The great healing]

122. "Träume. Unsere zweite Existenz," in *Musik und Medizin* **8**, 1981, pp. 17-35.
[Dreams. Our second life]

123. "Die Entwicklung der Psychotherapie im 20. Jahrhundert," in *Neue Zürcher Zeitung* **79**, May 5, 1981, pp. 69-70. Reprinted as "Abriß der Psychotherapie Entwicklung im 20.Jahrhundert," in *Von der Spannweite der Seele. Ausgewählte Vorträge und Aufsätze aus den Anwendungsbereichen des daseinsanalytischen Menschenverständnisses* (Bern: Benteli, 1982), pp. 182-198.
[The development of psychotherapy in the 20th Century]

[French translation: "Exposé sur le développement de la psychothérapie au 20e siècle," *Archives Suisses de Neurologie, Neurochirurgie et Psychiatrie* **128**(2), 1981, pp. 183-196. Reprinted as "Développement de la psychothérapie au 20e siècle," in *Psychiatrie Française* **14**(3), 1983, pp. 7-26].

124. "O inconsciente. Que è isso?" in *Tempo Psicanalítico* (Rio de Janeiro) **4**(1), 1981, pp. 28-40.
[The unconscious—What it is?]

[German translation: "Das Unbewußte—was ist es?" in *Von der Spannweite der Seele* (Bern: Huber, 1982), pp. 132-150].
[English translation: "The Unconscious—What Is It?," in *Review of Existential Psychology and Psychiatry* 20(1-3), 1986-1987, pp. 237-249. Reprinted in K. Hoeller (ed.), *Readings in Existential Psychology and Psychiatry* (Seattle: Review of Existential Psychology and Psychiatry, 1990), pp. 237-249.] (E.S. Goodstein)

125. "Die normale Angst," in *Neue Zürcher Zeitung* **271**, November 20-21, 1982, p. 37.
[Normal anxiety.]

126. "Zur Frage des sogenannten 'Stresses'," in *Zeitschrift der Klassisch Homöopathie* **27**(4), 1983, pp. 167-170.
[The question of so-called "stress"]

127. "Die Magie der psychosomatische Medizin," in *Psychosomatische Medizin* **11**(4) 1982, pp. 189-197.
[The magic of psychosomatic medicine] See 1985a.

128. "Gedanken zu Valerie Gampers Referat. An ihrer Sprache sollt ihr sie erkennen," in *Daseinsanalyse* **1**(1), 1984, pp. 58-65.
[Thoughts on Valerie Gampers' presentation. By their language shall you know them]

129. "Die Bedrängnis des Daseins," in *Rheinische Post* **303**, December 31, 1984, p. 2.
[The pressure of existence]

130. "Psychosomatische Medizin? Wissenschaft oder Magie?," in *Daseinsanalyse* **2**(2), 1985, pp. 107-119.
[Psychosomatic medicine. Science or magic?] See 1983b.

131. "Sonhar e psicoterapía," in *Revista de* Associação Brasileira de Daseinsanalyse (Sao Paulo) **6**, 1985, pp. 5-20.
[Dreaming and psychotherapy]

[German translation: "Woraus besteht der Mensch, wenn er träumt, un wo ist er dann?," in *Daseinsanalyse* **6**(3), 1989, pp. 149-160.]

[Note: An English version of the paper, "How and Where Are We When We Dream," was read at the University of Portland in 1989.]

132. **"After Thirty Years: Preface to A Psychiatrist Journeys to India (4th Edition, 1987)," in** *Review of Existential Psychiatry and Psychology* **27(1-3), 2002-2003, pp. 33-36. Reprinted as a monograph by K. Hoeller (ed.),** *The Heidegger-Boss Relationship* **(Seattle: Review of Existential Psychology and Psychiatry, 2008).** (Michael Eldred)
["After thirty years": Preface to *A Psychiatrist Journeys to India*]

133. "Daseinsanalytische Bemerkungen zum Wesen der Freudschen Psychoanalyse," in *Daseinsanalyse* **7**(3), 1990, pp. 167-173.
[Existential-analytical remarks on the nature of Freudian psychoanalysis]

134. **"Recent Considerations in Daseinsanalysis," in *The Humanistic Psychologist* 16(1), 1988, pp. 58-74.**
[Recent considerations in daseinsanalysis]

[Note: This is a transcription of a tape recordings of interviews with Erik Craig.]

135. **"Martin Heidegger Applied to Psychiatry and the Modern World" (1989), in *Review of Existential Psychology and Psychiatry* 27(1-3), 2002-2003, pp. 23-31. Reprinted as a monograph by K. Hoeller (ed.), *The Heidegger-Boss Relationship* (Seattle: Review of Existential Psychology and Psychiatry, 2008), pp. 23-31.** (Michael Eldred)
[Martin Heidegger applied to psychiatry and the modern world]

[Note: Lecture given at the Applied Heidegger Conference, Stanford University, September 8-10, 1989. According to Boss, the lecture was given at the University of California, Berkeley. See]

VI. CO-AUTHORED CONTRIBUTIONS

136. With G. Benedetti. "Psychoanalyse eines Sadisten," in *Psyche* **7**(5), 1953-54, pp. 241-263. Reprinted in *Von der Psychoanalyse zur Daseinsanalyse* (Vienna: Europaverlag, 1979), pp. 161-186. **"Psychoanalysis of a Sadist," in *Samiksha. Journal of the Indian Psychoanalytical Society* 7(1), 1953, pp. 18-38.**
[Psychoanalysis of a sadist]

[Czech translation: *Analyza Jednoho Sadisty* (Prague: Kabinet psychoterapie Psychiatrické kliniky fak. vseobec. lékarství, 1989)]

137. With H. Fierz-Monnier and A. Maeder. "Herkunft und Wesen des Archetypus-Begriffes. Ein Diskussion," in *Psyche* **7**(3), 1953, pp. 217-240.
[Origin and nature of the concept of the archetype. A discussion]

138. With G. Condrau. **"Existential Psychoanalysis,"** in B. Wolman (ed.), *Psychoanalytic Techniques* (New York: Basic Books, 1967), pp. 443-467. (B)
[Existential psychoanalysis]

139. With G. Condrau. **"Existential Analysis,"** in J.G. Howells (ed.), *Modern Perspectives in World Psychiatry* (London: Oliver & Boyd, 1968), pp. 488-518. (B)
[Existential analysis]

140. With G. Condrau. **"Daseinsanalysis,"** in W. Sahakian (ed.), *Psychopathology Today* (Itasca: Peacock, 1970), pp. 567-574. (B)
[Daseinsanalysis]

141. With A. Hicklin. "Daseinsanalyse," in *Lexikon der Psychologie* **1**, 1971, p. 347.
[Existential analysis]

142. With G. Condrau. "Die Daseinsanalyse in der Zürcher Psychiatrie von heute," in *Schweizer Archive der Neurologie, Neurochirurgie und Psychiatrie* **112**(1), 1973, pp. 21-30.
[Existential analysis in today's psychiatry in Zürich]

143. With G. Condrau. "Analyse existentielle (Daseinsanalyse)," in *Encyclopédie médico-chirurgicale* **5**, 1975, pp. 55-60. Reprinted as "Análisi existencial—Daseinsanalyse—Como a Daseinsanalyse entrou na Psiquiatria," in *Daseinsanalyse* (Sao Paulo) **2**, 1976, pp.5-23.
[Existential analysis (Daseinsanalysis)]

144. With B. Kenny. **"Phenomenological or Daseinsanalytic Approach,"** in J. Fosshage and C. Loew (eds.), *Dream Interpretation* (New York: SP Scientific Books, 1978; rev. ed., New York: PMA Publishing Corporation, 1987, pp. 149-189). (B)
[The phenomenological or existential-analytical approach]

145. With G. Condrau. "Die Weiterentwicklung der Daseinsanalyse nach Ludwig Binswanger," in U. Peters (ed.), *Die Psychologie des*

20.Jahrhunderts. Volume 10, *Ergebnisse für die Medizin* (Zürich: Kindler, 1980), pp. 728-739.
[The further development of Ludwig Binswanger's existential analysis]

146. With A. Holzhey-Kunz. "Das Phänomen des Widerstandes in der Daseinsanalyse," in H. Petzold (ed.), Widerstand - ein strittiges Konzept in der Psychotherapie (Paderborn: Jungfermann, 1981), pp. 173-189. Reprinted as "Das Konzept des Widerstandes in der Daseinsanalyse" in *Von der Spannweite der Seele. Ausgewählte Vorträge und Aufsätze aus den Anwendungsbereichen des daseinsanalytischen Menschenverständnisses* (Bern: Benteli, 1982), pp. 111-131.
[The phenomenon of resistance in existential analysis]

147. With D. Rhee. **"Dialogue Between Prof. Medard Boss and Prof. Dongshick Rhee" [June 12 and June 15, 1976]**, in 精神治療 *[Psychotherapy]* (Seoul) 6, 1996, pp. 30-43. Transcribed from audio tape recordings of two interviews, online: http://taopsychotherapy.org/rhee/02_en_sub_view.php?no=15&rno=&page=1&search1=&search2=&table_mode=rhee_papers and http://www.taopsychotherapy.org/rhee/02_en_sub_view.php?no=14&rno=&page=1&search1=&search2=&table_mode=rhee_papers
[Dialogues with Dongshick Rhee]

148. With M. Boss-Linsmayer and M. Groth. "An International Bibliography of the Writings of Medard Boss 1929-2002," in *Review of Existential Psychology and Psychiatry* 27(1-3), 2002-2003, pp. 155-171, reprinted in a monograph by K. Hoeller (ed.), *The Heidegger-Boss Relationship* (Seattle: Review of Existential Psychology and Psychiatry, 2008), pp. 155-171.
[An international bibliography pf the writings of Medard Boss 1929-2003] (first iteration)

VII. AUDIO RECORDING

149. "Ein neues Traumverständnis und seine praktisch-therapeutischen Anwendungsmöglichkeiten" [1976], in *Sonderedition anläßlich der 50. Lindauer Psychotherapiewoche 2000: Bedeutende Vorträge aus den Jahren 1970 - 1996* (Schwarzach: Auditorium Verlag, 2001). [Audio recording.]
[A new understanding of dreams and its possibilities in practical therapeutic application]

VIII. MISCELLANEOUS

150. **Letters to Erna M. Hoch (1960).** Erna M. Hoch, *Sources and Resources. A Western Psychiatrist's Search for Meaning in the Ancient Indian Scriptures* (Zürich: Rüegger, 1991): "Messenger between East and West," pp. 251-253 [March 12, 1960], 263 and 281 [April 10, 1960], and 282 [May 22, 1960].
[Letters to Erna Hoch]

151. "Ist menschliche Schuld psychotherapeutisch heilbar?" at the Katholische Akademie Freiburg, June 3, 1984. Unpublished lecture.
[Is human guilt curable with psychotherapy?]

AWARDS

1959 Honorary Member, Indian Psychiatric Society (Lucknow).
1962 Corresponding Member, Royal College of Psychiatrists of Great Britain (London).
1967 Honorary President, International Federation for Medical Psychotherapy (Zürich).
1969 Honorary Member, Swiss Medical Society for Psychotherapy (Zürich).
1971 Recipient, Great Therapist Award, American Psychological Association (Washington).

1971 Honorary Member, Swiss Society of Psychosomatic Medicine (Zürich).
1972 Honorary Member, Ibero-Latin American Psychiatric Society (Buenos Aires).
1975 Honorary President, Brazilian Association of Existential Analysis (Sao Paulo).
1982 Honorary Guest, Twelfth International Congress of Psychotherapy (Rio de Janeiro).
1985 Honorary President, Swiss Society for Daseinsanalysis (Zürich).
1988 Recipient, Margrit Egnër Prize (University of Zürich).

CHRONOLOGICAL LIST OF PUBLICATIONS[1]

1929 [On the question of the evolutionary biological significance of alcohol]

1931 [Psychological and characterological investigations of antisocial psychopaths using the Rorschach Inkblot Test]

1933 [Hallucinations in process of formation]

1935a [Psychic energy displacements in the course of a schizophrenic episode]

1935b [The psychodynamics of the sleep cure in schizophrenics]

1936 [Indications and effects of the "sleep cure"]

1937 [Historical review of the fundamental principles of the therapy of schizophrenia]

1938a [Preparation of individuals with severe chronic schizophrenia for group occupational therapy]

1938b [The psychopathology of dreams in schizophrenic and organic psychoses]

1939 [On three categories of avoidable failures in general medical practice]

1940a [Brief and intensive psychotherapy]

---

1 Italicized items are books. Bolded items have been translated into English or first appeared in English. For those already translated I have provided my own preferred translation as given at the end of each entry in square brackets above. The titled of those published first in English are given as Boss published them.

1940b [On the hidden challenges to psychological well-being and their reduction]
1940c [*Physical illness as a result of psychological imbalance*]
1941a [Functional disturbances of sleep in schizophrenia]
1941b [Food rationing and popular psychology]
1941c [Psychological health on the front lines (military psychiatry)]
1941d [Early and recent electroshock therapies and electroshock therapists]
1943 [*The significance of psychology for human relationships and community life*]
1944a [The function of the psychiatric counseling center in independent army units]
1944b [*The shape of marriage and its forms of disintegration. A contribution to the psychopathology of the formation of human community life*]
1945 [Bed-wetting]
1947 [**Meaning and content of sexual perversions. An existential-analytical contribution to the psychopathology of the phenomenon of love**]
1948a [The method and goal of depth-psychological therapy]
1948b [The possibilities and limits of psychotherapy]
1949 [Blood pressure ailments as a human problem]

1950a [Fundamentals of psychosomatic medicine]
1950b [Reply to the report on my presentation at the 66th gathering of Southwest German psychiatrists and neurologists held in Badenweiler (Conference on the Boss-Mitscherlich controversy)] See 1981a.
1950c [Latest advances in the field of psychoanalysis]
1951a [Contribution on the existential-analytical foundation of psychiatric thinking]
1951b [Experiences with the hypnotic Plexonal [Sopolamine] (Sandoz)]
1952a [**Man and technology in today's medicine**]
1952b [The significance of existential analysis for psychology and psychiatry]
1953a [On the origin and essence of the depth-psychological concept of the archetype]

1953b [How should frigidity be evaluated and treated in practice?]
1953c [Regulation of the activity of non-medical psychologists]
1953d [*The dream and its interpretation*]
1953e [Origin and nature of the concept of the archetype. A discussion] With H. Fierz-Monnier and A. Maeder.
1953f **[Psychoanalysis of sadist]** With G. Benedetti.
1954a [*Introduction to psychosomatic medicine*] See 1978c.
1954b [Basics of the scientific nature of dream interpretation]
1955a [*Third internation congress of psychotherapy*] (ed.) With H. Fierz and B. Stokvis.
1955b [Psychosomatic medicine in distress]
1956a **[Moreno's 'Existentialism, Daseinanalyse and Psychodrama': A Discussion]**
1956b **[Analytics of existence and psychotherapy. On the limits of psychoanalysis]**
1957a [*Psychoanalysis and the analytics of existence*]
1957b **[A Psychotherapeutic contribution to the theory of schizophrenia]**
1957c [The mechanism of action and indications for psychotherapy]
1957d [Summary and closing remarks at the international symposium on the psychotherapy of schizophrenia (Lausanne 1957)]
1959a [*A psychiatrist's journey to India*] See 1987.
1959b [Martin Heidegger and the doctors]
1959c [Psychotherapy for the practicing physician]
1959d [Brief and intensive psychotherapy for essential hypertension]
1959e [Psychoanalysis and the analytics of 'existence"]

1960a **[Letter to Heidegger, January 12, 1960)]**
1960b [The intensive psychotherapy of psychosomatic diseases]
1960c **[The I? Motivation?]**
1960d **[Letters to Erna M. Hoch]**
1960-1961a [Existential-analytical remarks on Freud's concept of the 'unconscious']
1960-1961b [The significance of existential analysis for psychoanalytic practice]
1961a **[Psychosomatics and existentialism]**
1961b **[Why does man behave socially at all?]**
1962a **[Outline of the analysis of** Dasein]

1962b [**The conception of man in natural science and existential analysis**]
1962c [*Fear of life, feelings of guilt, and psychotherapeutic liberation*]
1963 [Thoughts on a schizophrenic hallucination]
1965a [**President's opening address, August 24, 1964. VIth International congress of psychotherapy**]
1965b [**President's closing address, August 29, 1964. VIth International Congress of Psychotherapy**]
1965c [**Discussion of Ruesch, August 24, 1964**]
1965d [Encounter in psychotherapy]
1965e [**Preface to C. Seguin,** The doctor and his patient]
1966a [Five introductory lectures on the analytics of existence]
1966b [Evidence for the influence of psychotherapy on the religious attitude of the analysand]
1967a [Demythologization of psychosomatic medicine]
1967b [Paradigm and counterparadigm in psychosomatic medicine]
1967c [**Existential psychoanalysis**] With G. Condrau.
1968a [**Conversation with Mary Harrington Hall**]
1968b [**Existential analysis**] With G. Condrau.
1968-1969 [Man—an object of science]

1970a [A needed revolution in medical thinking]
1970b [**Daseinsanalysis**] With G. Condrau.
1970c [Foreword to *Govind Amrit*]
1971a [*Outline of medicine and psychology. Approaches to a phenomenological physiology, psychology, pathology, therapy and to an existential preventative medicine*]
1971b [A needed revolution in worldview]
1971c [Daseinsanalyse] With A. Hicklin.
1972a [**The training of the future psychotherapist. Improvement of psychiatric services and teaching programs**]
1972b [Warning signs of a storm in psychology and psychiatry. Epilogue to a revolutionary international congress on psychotherapy]
1972c [The physician and death. An existential analytic investigation]
1973a [**Medard Boss**]
1973b [The significance of daseinsanalysis for psychiatry illustrated by the treatment of a schizophrenic psychosis]

1973c [Sigmund Freud and natural scientific method of thinking]
1973d [Daseinsanalysis in today's psychiatry in Zürich] With G. Condrau.
1974a [Corresponding changes in quality of social life and forms of neurosis in the 20th century]
1974b [Psycho-somatic medicine and the principle of causaility]
1975a [Solitude and community]
1975b [*It dreamt me last night...*]
1975c [The schizophrenic's "being ill" understood in terms of existential analysis]
1975d [Existential analysis (Daseinsanalysis)] With G. Condrau.
1976a [**Dreams and the dreamed from the existential analytic perspective**]
1976b [**Flight from death—mere survival; and flight into death—suicide**]
1976c [Culture and psychotherapy]
1976d [A new understanding of dreams and its possibilities in practical therapeutic application] (audio recording)
1976f [The mind-body problem in light of daseinsanalysis]
1977a [The ontogenesis of man... from the perspective of the daseinsanalyst]
1977b [The existential approach and psychotherapeutic suggestibility in human physical ailments]
1977c [The psychotherapeutic process]
1977d [**Thanks to Martin Heidegger. A note on his Zollikon seminars**]
1977e [**Existential analysis**]
1977f [*Being alive and living life*]
1977g [Education—Yes or no?]
1977h [Envy triggers terror. The phenomenon of human violence]
1977i [Living with terror]
1977j [Medard Boss [Tribute to Martin Heidegger]
1978a [Contradiction contradicted]
1978b [Current changes in the identification of the neuroses in psychotherapy]
1978c [*Practice of psychosomatics. Illness and personal fate*] See 1954a.

1978d [**The phenomenological or Daseinsanalytic approach**] With B. Kenny.
1979a [Being-towards-death from the perspective of depth psychology]
1979b [**The irrational in psychotherapeutic practice**]
1979c [*From psychoanalysis to daseinsanalysis. Paths to a new self-understanding*]
1979d [Sexuality and psychotherapy]

1980a [Martin Heidegger and his significance for the evolution of society]
1980b [Dreaming. The great healing]
1980c [The further development of Ludwig Binswanger's daseinsanalysis] With G. Condrau.
1981a [Closing remarks (Conference on the Boss-Mitscherlich controversy)] See 1950b.
1981b [Dreams. Our second life]
1981c [The development of psychotherapy in the 20th Century]
1981d [**The unconscious—What it is?**]
1981e [The phenomenon of resistance in daseinsanalysis] With A. Holzhey-Kunz.
1981f [Encounter and self-confrontation in guilt and in conscience]
1981g [The world of drives and personalization]
1981h [Anxiety and composure from the existential analytic perspective]
1982a [Normal anxiety.]
1982b [*On the wingspan of the soul. Selected lectures and essays from areas of application of the existential analytic understanding of man*]
1982c [Actuality as the self-revelation of what is there]
1982d [**A phenomenological approach to sexual perversions**]
1982e [The existential analytic interpretation of dreams]
1983a [The question of so-called "stress"]
1983b [The magic of psychosomatic medicine]
1984a [Thoughts on Valerie Gampers' presentation. By their language shall you know them]
1984b [The pressure of existence]
1984c [Is human guilt curable with psychotherapy?]

1985a [Psychosomatic medicine. Science or magic?]
1985b [The magic of psychosomatic medicine]
1985c [Dreaming and psychotherapy]
1987 [**After thirty years: Preface to *A psychiatrist journeys to India* (4th Edition)**] See 1957a.
1988 [**Recent considerations in daseinsanalysis**]
1989a [**Martin Heidegger, *Zollikon seminars: Protocols, conversations, letters* (ed.)**]
1989b [**Martin Heidegger applied to psychiatry and the modern world**]

1990a [Existential analytic remarks on the nature of Freudian psychoanalysis]
1990b [**Preface to the American Translation of Martin Heidegger's *Zollikon Seminars***]
1991 [Martin Heidegger's initiatives for a different kind of psychiatry]
1996 [**Dialogues with Dongshick Rhee**]

2001 [Preface to Martin Heidegger, *Zollikon Seminars. Protocols—Conversations—Letters*]
2002/2003 [**An International Bibliography of the Writings of Medard Boss 1929-2002**] (first iteration)

Thematic Index to the Chronological List of Publications

anxiety
1981h, 1982a

archetypes
1953b, 1953e

da-seinanalysis [*Daseinsanalyse*]
(existential analysis)
1951a,1952b, 1962a, 1962b, 1966a, 1968b,
1970b, 1971c, 1973d, 1974b, 1975d, 1977e,
1978d, 1979c, 1988

death
1972a, 1976b, 1979a

dreams
1938b, 1953d, 1954b, 1975b, 1976a, 1976d
[audio recording], 1980b, 1981b, 1982e,
1985c, 1989c

ECT
1941c

enuresis
1945

existential psychoanalysis
1967c

frigidity
1953b

hallucinations
1933, 1963

hypertension
1949

India
1959a, 1987

lay psychoanalysis
1953c

medicine
1970a, 1971a

mind-body problem
1976f

motivation
1960c

paraphilias (perversions)
1931, 1947, 1953f, 1982d

pharmacotherapy
1951b

phenomenology
1978e, 1982d

psychoanalysis
1948a, 1950c, 1956b, 1957a,
1959e,1960/61b, 1990a

psychodrama
1956b

psychosomatic medicine
1940c, 1949, 1950a, 1954a, 1955b, 1960b,
1961a, 1967a, 1974b, 1977b,1978c, 1983b,
1985b

psychotherapy
1940a, 1948a, 1948b, 1957c, 1959c,1959d,
1962c, 1965d, 1966b, 1972a, 1972b, 1976c,
1977c, 1978b, 1979b, 1979d, 1981c, 1981e,
1985, 1996

resistance
1981e

Thematic Index to the Chronological List of Publications

Rorschach test
1931

schizophrenia
1933, 1935a, 1935b, 1937, 1938a, 1938b,
1941c, 1957b, 1963 1973b, 1975c

social psychology
1943, 1944b, 1961b, 1974a, 1975a

somatic therapy
1941d, 1951b

spirituality
1966b

stress
1983a

suicide
1976b

technology
1952a

unconscious, the
1960/61a, 1981d

Name Index to the Chronological List of Publications

Binswanger, Ludwig
1980c

Boss, Medard
1968a, 1973a

Freud, Sigmund
1973c

Heidegger, Martin
1959b, 1960a, 1977d, 1977j, 1980a,
1989a,1989b, 1990b, 1991, 2001

Hoch, Erna
1960d

Kaul, Govind
1970c

Moreno, Jacob
1956a

Rhee, Dongshick
1976e

Seguín, Carlos
1965e

Glossary

Analyse	analysis (taking apart), as in *Psychoanalyse, Existenzanalyse* and *Daseinsanalyse*
Analytik	analytics (a distinguishing of elements within a whole structure)
analytisch	analytic (referring to *Analyse* or *Analytik*)
Dasein	existence
Daseinsanalyse	existential analysis
daseinsanalytisch	existential-analytic
Daseinsanalytik	analytics of existence
daseinsanalytisch	existential-analytical
daseinsgemäße	existentially informed
daseinsgemäßig	existentially-informed
existentiell	existentialist
Existenz	existing
Existenzanalyse	analysis of existing
Existenzial	existentive (an element of the structure of the be[ing] of existence)
existenzial	existentive (pertaining to the Existenzials)
existenziale Analytik	existentive analytics (Heidegger's project in *Sein und Zeit*)
Existenzphilosophie	philosophy of existing
existieren	to ek-sist
existiert	ek-sists
realiter existiert	is really there (in Holzhey-Kunz)

Glossary

Existieren	ek-sisting
Sein	be[-ing] or [to-]be
Seiende	what is there (all there is); an instance of what is there
Zu-sein	to-being (to-ness)

Index

An overview of my translation decisions is given in the Glossary (pp. 247-248). The Bibliography is followed by two indices (pp. 244-246) keyed to a chronological list of Boss's writings (pp. 237-243) detailed in the Bibliography.

I. Topics

analysis of existing
  (*Existenzanalyse*) 13-19
analytics of existence
  (*Daseinsanalytik*) 19-21, 26n, 27, 30, 33, 36-38, 40-42, 52, 55-60, 79, 81, 123, 149, 152
anthropology 19, 39, 50, 52, 103
anxiety (*Angst*) 150, 152-153

being (*Sein*) 109, 114n, 115
being-with (*Mitsein*) 79
boredom 80, 83, 94

clearing (*Lichtung*) 121-122
co-existence (*Mit-dasein*) 120, 124-125
concern (*Fürsorge*) (see "looking after")
consciousness (*Bewußtsein*) 43, 82, 91
cybernetics 77, 81

da-seinanalysis 7, 54, 94, 123-127
Daseinsanalysis 21n, 36, 54, 107-108
dreams 61-65

ego 10, 35, 40, 43
ego psychology 34
ek-sisting (*Existieren*) 18, 20, 150, 151
existence (*Dasein*) 1, 10, 15, 17-20, 21n, 22, 26n, 32n, 33, 35, 38, 39, 40, 52, 55, 59, 103, 108-109, 114, 116n, 118-120, 125-126, 149, 150, 151, 152n, 153

existential analysis (*Daseinsanalyse*) 1, 4-5, 7n, 10-11, 12, 14, 19, 21n, 22-23, 27, 29, 33, 36-37, 41-42, 48, 53n, 54, 58-61, 64, 75, 91, 97-98, 104-105, 107, 113n, 116, 119-120, 123-124, 129, 149
existential psychoanalysis (*psychanalyse existentielle*) 21
existential psychotherapy 3-4, 12, 18, 30
existentialism 3, 27n, 37, 59
existentive (*Existenzial*) 26n, 37n
existing (*Existenz*) 13-22, 26n, 55, 59, 125-126, 150, 152n

fundamental ontology
  (*Fundamentalontologie*) 20, 26n, 36-37, 103, 112-113, 120, 126, 150-151

Hindu philosophy 91, 99, 101-103, 109-110, 112, 113, 115-116, 126
humanistic psychology (Third Force) 4, 14, 18, 34n, 69

illumination (*Lichtung*) 11, 106, 107n, 108, 114
interventional looking after
  (*einspringende Fürsorge*) 10, 89

logotherapy 13-16, 19, 125
looking after (*Fürsorge*) 10, 89, 120
love 25, 31-35, 42, 48-49, 149, 151-152n, 153

[249]

Index

medicine 8, 45n, 66-69, 102n, 103, 203

ontology 20, 27n, 39

perversions (paraphilias) 25-50
phenomenology 3, 15, 19, 40-41, 67, 80, 150
philosophy of existing (*Existenzphilosophie*) 13, 15, 18-19, 26n,
psychiatry 1, 5-9, 22, 27-28, 32n, 33, 34n, 40-43, 52n, 66-69, 74, 80, 102, 104-105, 114
psychoanalysis 1-4, 7-11, 15, 18, 21-22, 27-29, 39, 44, 52, 55-56, 58, 68, 71, 78-79, 102, 106, 123, 129, 203
psychosomatics 67, 81, 202
psychotherapy 1-7, 10, 12-21, 37, 52-53, 59, 64, 66, 68, 72n, 96, 102, 104, 120, 129

schizophrenia 7, 29, 80, 125
stress 81, 96
symbolic value 45, 49, 52

technology 71, 81, 99-100, 108, 114
there-being (*Da-sein*) 54, 109, 121-122n
therapeut 11n, 99, 103-105, 120, 124-126
therapy/therapeutic situation 1-8, 9-11, 39, 44n, 60, 66-67n, 68-72n, 89, 94, 97-98, 104-106, 119-121, 123-129

unconscious (*Unbewußt*) 34-35, 45

way-making looking after (*vorausspringende Fürsorge*) 10, 89 120
what is there (*das Seiende*) 19, 21n, 91, 114

Zen Buddhism 111, 113-116, 126

II. Names

Allport, Gordon 34n, 69

Beaufret, Jean 20
Behn-Eschenburg, Hans 28
Berg, Jan Hendrik van den 4-7
Bernfeld, Siegfried 28
Binswanger, Ludwig 4, 10, 12, 19, 27-28
Blankenburg, Wolfgang 96
Bleuler, Eugen vi, 28
Bleuler, Manfred 96
Boss, Medard vi, 7-8, 84-85, 99-129, 202-204
Boss-Linsmayer, Marianne 85-86, 204
Buber, Martin 81, 95
Bugental, James 6

Condrau, Gion 47, 48n

Ellenberger, Henri 30, 54
Erikson, Erik 5

Frankl, Viktor 12, 19
Freud, Sigmund vi, 2, 4-6, 10, 18-19, 21-22n, 26n, 28-29, 33, 34n, 39, 43-44, 56, 59, 62, 64, 71n, 72n, 75, 78-79, 82, 90-91, 103-107, 123, 150, 152n

Gebsattel, Viktor von 44-52, 79, 91
Goldstein, Kurt 29
Groth, Miles 44n, 67n, 72n, 119n, 204n

Heidegger, Hermann 85-86
Heidegger, Martin v-vi, 2-3, 7, 9-11, 16-22, 24-96, 97-116, 120-129
Herrmann, Friedrich-Wilhelm von 78, 83, 86, 89
Hoch, Erna 87n, 88, 93, 110, 113-114
Holzhey-Kunz, Alice 10, 12, 16-23, 29n
Husserl, Edmund 2, 40-41, 43, 80, 91, 150

Jaspers, Karl 19, 26n
Jung, Carl Gustav vi, 6, 29, 62, 105, 107
Jünger, Ernst 80

Kaul, Govind 114n, 116n, 118-121
Kayande, J.M. 116n, 120-121
Kierkegaard, Søren 19
Krafft-Ebing, Wilhelm von 32

Längle, Alfried 12-16, 19-21
Laing, R.D. 1, 4-7

Index

Marcuse, Herbert 82
May, Rollo 6, 56, 69
Merleau-Ponty, Maurice 2

Pandey, Kanti Chandra 113-114

Richardson, William J. 54, 84-85
Rogers, Carl 19

Sartre, Jean-Paul 2-3, 26n, 37
Shankaracharya, Adi 79n, 91, 116
Szasz, Thomas 6, 32n

Trawny, Peter 70-96

Weizsäcker, Carl Friedrich von 80
Weizsäcker, Viktor von 91
Wiener, Norbert 81